# A Digger's Guide To Medicinal Plants

## 2nd Edition

Text by
Allen Lockard and Alice Q. Swanson

Photographs by
Alice Q. Swanson

### Dedication

To Willard Magee
Teacher and Friend

### And in memory of

Dwayne Triplett
Partner and Friend

American Botanicals
Eolia, Missouri
2004

For information about permission
to reproduce selections from this book, write to:

American Botanicals
P.O. Box 158 • Rt. FF
Eolia, Missouri 63344

Library of Congress Control Number: 2004102355

ISBN 0-9663398-2-7

Printed in the United States of America

American Botanicals, PO Box 158 • Rt. FF
Eolia, Missouri 63344

# Introduction

Before the United States was the United States, country folks were harvesting roots and herbs from the wild. While some of these plants were used to make home medicines, the majority were sold to companies who exported the plants to Europe and Asia. Many families made part of their living each year gathering and digging roots and herbs. Even some frontier scouts, surveyors, and fur trappers supplemented their incomes by digging. Old records show that Daniel Boone dug Ginseng and sold it to a company in Philadelphia for export to China.

Today the harvesting and digging of medicinal plants and roots continues to provide an income for many rural families. Those whose livelihoods depend on income from these plants generally employ sound harvesting practices, often learned from their parents or grandparents. Indeed, some diggers have even harvested in patches of Goldenseal or Ginseng that their fathers or grandfathers once harvested. Wise wildcrafting practices do not harm plant populations.

There are people who voice fears that the continued harvesting of plants from the wild threatens their existence. That may be so in some situations. It cannot be denied that some diggers harvest thoughtlessly, dig out of season, and ignore the traditional wisdom of leaving at least 10% of any plant colony to reseed and reproduce. However, even with this ruthless treatment some seeds and roots will often be left behind. If left to Mother Nature's care, these survivors will produce a new patch.

A more overwhelming threat to these plants is the increasing destruction of their habitat. Diggers find that those areas that have been sprayed with herbicides or other poisons, and areas that have been clear-cut or bulldozed for development, can no longer be harvested. Once a forest has been clear-cut or a hollow bulldozed, the growing conditions needed by wild plants will have been destroyed. There is then little chance that the plants will grow there again. Herbicides sprayed on pastures, roadsides, and right of ways destroy plant populations. Where plants do survive, they contain harmful residues and should not be harvested for human consumption.

With the increasing demand for medicinal plants and the increasing prices paid for them, more and more people are looking to the woods for an additional source of income. To insure that there will be a continuing supply of wild medicinal plants, certain conservation practices need to be followed by those harvesting them. It is our hope that this book will serve as a practical guide to those new to harvesting as well as those who continue a family tradition.

It is also our hope that you will consider cultivating some of the plants we have included in this guide. A wood lot planted to Goldenseal this year can produce its first crop of roots in three years. A small field planted to Catnip can produce its first crop next year. Cultivating medicinal herbs can take stress off wild populations and can also insure you of a continuing source of harvest.

Medicinal plants have been used by millions of people for thousands of years to treat and prevent illness. With the continuing loss of natural habitat for these plants, it is more important than ever that we harvest with great care and begin to grow these plants ourselves. Good wildcrafting practices and cultivation preserve the plant populations and the digger's future source of income. These practices also insure that there will continue to be medicinal plants for our children and grandchildren to use.

# What, When, Where, and How

Harvesting medicinal plant material for the commercial market is hard work. Locating, harvesting, cleaning, and drying roots and plant material take time, thought, common sense, and effort. Because the medicinal plants you harvest are intended for human consumption, certain guidelines need to be followed to insure purity and potency.

Wise harvesting and reseeding of medicinal plants will provide future harvests. Following are some general guidelines for conservation practices and for harvesting, cleaning, drying, and preparing plants for market. More specific information can be found in this guide under the entries for individual plants.

## General Guidelines

✦ **Be sure you know for certain the plant you are harvesting.** Study the pictures and descriptions in this guide or other plant books. Ask friends who also dig and harvest. If you are not absolutely sure, dig or gather a few roots or leaves of the plant and take it to your buyer for positive identification.

✦ **Obey all Federal, State, and Local Laws regarding harvesting of plants.** Ask your State Plant Board, State Agricultural Department, or county agricultural agent for their guidelines and laws. In most states you will need a permit to gather from state or national forest lands.

✦ **Do not trespass.** Ask permission from property owners before going on their land.

✦ **Collect medicinal plants where they are reasonably abundant and grow vigorously.** If a plant is uncommon in your area, or if there are just a few, leave them. The plant probably grows elsewhere in abundance and will be better harvested from that area.

✦ **Never dig or collect all the plants in an area.** If you selectively harvest a patch of Ginseng, Goldenseal, or most other medicinal roots, you will be able to return to that patch again and again. Dig the older, more mature plants and leave the younger, smaller plants for future harvesting. Digging of the older plants aerates the soil and gives the smaller plants room to spread their roots and grow more vigorously. When gathering herbs like Skullcap or Passion Flower, leave at least 10% of each patch to set seeds. This will insure future health and growth of the patch.

✦ **Rotate your patches.** Locate two or three patches and then rotate your harvesting. It is best not to harvest from the same patch two years in a row.

✦ **Harvest roots and plant material at the appropriate time of the year.** There are state and local laws that protect certain plants. For example, Wild American Ginseng has a controlled harvest season in all 19 states where it grows. This time varies from state to state, and sometimes from year to year. Check with your state plant board, county agricultural agent, or your buyer for information on your local Ginseng season and any other laws or guidelines regarding the proper time for harvesting of wild plants in your state.

✦ **Never harvest plants that are on the threatened or endangered species list.** Your state plant board, county agriculture agent, or buyer will be able to provide you with a list of these plants.

## When To Harvest

Because the plant material you dig or gather is used in medicinal products, harvest roots and herbs when the plants are richest in medicinal properties. Contact your state plant agencies or talk to your buyer for information to determine when this time is in your area.

### Roots

The *root* of a plant is the part that exists below the surface of the soil and serves to bring food and water from the soil to the plant. Root structures may consist of taproots, rhizomes, corms, or tubers accompanied by smaller rootlets and hair roots.

Roots of perennial plants are most often harvested in the fall, when plant growth has stopped and seeds have matured. At this time the root is richest in its medicinal quality. Harvesting roots before the seeds have set will threaten the health and regeneration of the plant population. Roots can be harvested through the winter months, but should not be harvested once the sap begins to rise and the plant begins to put out new growth.

Roots dug in the spring or early summer contain more water, are more difficult to dry, and weigh less when dried than those dug in the fall. They also contain less of the medicinal qualities desired by those using the roots. If the quality of the root being dug is inferior, buyers will look elsewhere for their supply.

Be sure to replant seeds and replace the soil in the holes after removing the roots from the ground.

**Herbs and Leaves**

The above ground parts of a plant — the stem, leaves, flowers, and fruit — constitute the *herb*.

Harvest herbs just as the plant begins to flower. This is the time the plant is richest in medicinal qualities. When harvesting herbs, do not pull on the plants. Cut them off, and leave the root system intact in the ground for re-growth. Leave at least 10% of each patch to set seeds for future growth and harvesting.

Gather leaves when they are fully mature. Take care not to excessively damage the plant, tree, or its branches. Pruning after harvest will encourage heavier re-growth for the next season.

The best time to harvest leaves and herbs is on sunny days in the late morning, after the dew has dried.

## Barks

The outer skin, or *bark* of a tree, is most easily removed in the spring and early summer when the sap is rising. Harvest from the branches of the trees rather than the trunk. Strip bark from one side of branches only. **Never girdle the trunk or the branches**. Girdling is stripping the bark away from the trunk or a branch all the way around. Girdling the trunk will kill a tree.

Both tree bark and root bark are harvested from some trees. Root bark stops at the top of the soil; above that point is tree bark.

Strip bark from trees in areas where they are going to be logged or bulldozed. **Do not gather bark from dead trees**.

## Cleaning, Drying, and Preparing for Market

### Roots

Immediately after digging, shake all loose dirt from roots and remove all stems. Rinse the roots in running water, removing loose dirt with your fingers. Continue rinsing until the water runs away clear. Do not scrub roots with a brush or use soap to clean them. Shake excess water from the roots, and spread them out in single layers on screens or cardboard flats.

Air dry roots out of the sun in a well ventilated area. If drying outdoors, protect roots from the dew in the evening and morning.

**Never use an oven, microwave, wood stove, hot tin roof, or the back of your car to dry roots.** When dried this way roots will appear dark and roasted in color and have no medicinal or monetary value. Most roots will dry whole in a warm, dry place that gets good air circulation. A well ventilated attic is a good place. Large roots like Butterfly Weed and Missouri Snake Root will dry more quickly if split.

**Never split or string Ginseng.** Be careful to keep Ginseng roots intact. Broken roots lose their value.

When roots are thoroughly dry, store them in paper or burlap bags. **Never bag a root until it is completely dry, and do not store in plastic bags.** Plastic causes the roots to sweat and mold. Never mix green or wet roots with dry ones. The dry roots will absorb moisture from the green, and the whole crop will be ruined.

11

## Herbs and Leaves

Pick through leaves and herbs and remove all foreign matter that may have become entangled in them. Remove any dead leaves. Air dry leaves and herbs out of the sun on drying racks in single layers, turning them occasionally. If left in the sun, the plant material will shrivel and turn brown, rather than dry. Most leaves should retain their green color. If drying out of doors, protect them from the dew in the evenings and early mornings.

Never bag herbs or leaves until they are thoroughly dry. Never mix wet herbs and leaves with dry ones. Any moisture can cause the herb to mold if it is shut off from the air. Store dried herbs and leaves in paper or burlap bags. **Never bag dried herbs in plastic bags.** Plastic can cause leaves and herbs to scald and turn black. Molded or scalded leaves and herbs have no medicinal or monetary value.

## Barks

Dry bark as you do herbs and leaves, on racks out of the sun. To test bark for dryness, press the inner bark with your thumbnail. If any moisture comes to the surface, the bark is not thoroughly dry.

As with medicinal roots and plant material, store thoroughly dry bark in paper bags or burlap.

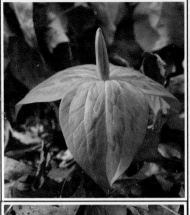
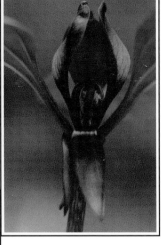
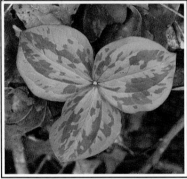

# Bethroot
*Trillium erectum*

**Also Called:**  Red Trillium, Purple Trillium, Birthroot, Wake Robin, Stinking Benjamin

**Description:**  Bethroot is a perennial plant growing to 2 feet in height with a single stem, a whorl of three leaves, and a single flower that blooms at the center of the whorl.

*Leaves:*  Three broad leaves in a whorl grow near the top of the

13

slender stem. The leaves are oval, almost as broad as they are long and narrowing at the base. They are a rich green and sometimes show patches of a darker green.

*Flowers:* At the top of the stem a solitary 3-petaled flower blooms. The flowers are a deep red to maroon in color with three greenish sepals. The flower gives off an unpleasant fishy odor.

*Roots:* Roots are oblong and tuberous with fine lines of circles or rings at the top and the marks of past stems. It is a light brown externally and yellowish within.

**Where:** Bethroot grows in shady woods and ravines in rich moist soils. It ranges from Canada south to Tennessee, Missouri, and Arkansas.

**What:** Harvest the root. Be sure to check with your local plant board or county agriculture agent to confirm that this is not on the threatened or endangered species list in your area.

**When:** Dig root in the fall after the plant has set its seed.

**How:** See Pages 10-11 for general guidelines

on cleaning, drying, and preparing roots for market.

**Uses:** Native Americans used the root to east the pains of childbirth, regulate menstrual flow, and to alleviate meno-pausal discomforts. It was also used for bronchial and lung problems including asthma and for hemorrhages.

## Notes

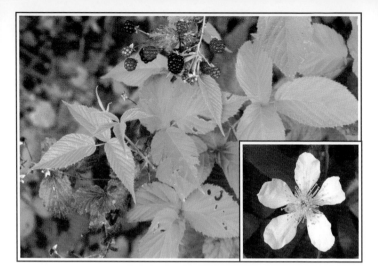

# Blackberry
*Rubus occidentalis*

**Also Called:**  Brambleberry, Dewberry, Black Raspberry

**Description:**  These shrubby perennial bushes are often found growing in thick patches. Blackberry bushes have arching canes that are lined with numerous curved, sharp thorns.

*Leaves:*  Leaves are sharply toothed and are found in groups of threes. The underside of the leaves have a whitish sheen to them.

*Flowers:*  An abundance of white

flowers, similar in appearance to wild roses, appear along the canes in clusters. They bloom from April to July.

*Fruit:*  Fruit is red before it ripens into deep blue-black. Berries ripen in late June to July and continue ripening into the early fall.

**Where:**  Blackberry patches can be found in old fields, meadows, thickets, pastures, and along fence rows and roadsides throughout the United States. Many people think blackberries are invasive weeds and may be more than willing to let you dig them out.

**What:**  Harvest the roots.

**When:**  Harvest roots in the fall or before new growth begins in the spring.

**How:**  See Page 10-11 for general guidelines on cleaning, drying, and preparing roots for market.

**Uses:**  Blackberry roots have been traditionally used for diarrhea, dysentery, wounds, and as a female tonic.

## Notes

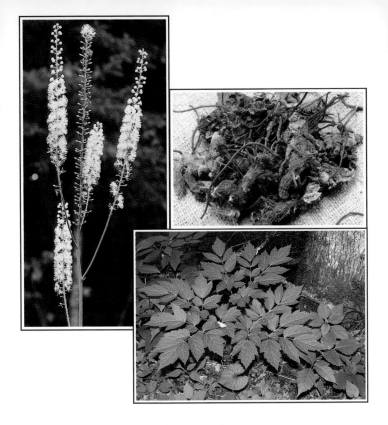

# Black Cohosh
*Cimicifuga racemosa*

**Also Called:**  Bugbane, Papoose Root, Squawroot, Rattlesnake Root, Rattle-top

**Description:**  Black Cohosh is a tall, impressive perennial plant that looks like a shrub. It can grow to a height of 9 feet or more.

*Leaves:* Leaves are composed of 2 to 5 leaflets that have toothed edges. The leafy bottom part of the plant can grow up to 6 feet in height.

*Flowers:* A slender stem rises from the shrubby base 3 feet or more and is topped by 2 to 3 spikes of white, plume-like flowers. The plant flowers from June to September. Seed pods follow the flower and stay on the plant into the winter. These pods are thick and dry and seeds rattle in them when the winter winds blow.

*Roots:* The root is large and knotty with knobby bumps or scars where past stems have grown. Freshly dug roots are a dark reddish brown in color on the outside and white inside.

**Where:** Black Cohosh grows in rich open woods and at the edges of dense woods. It ranges from Southern Ontario across to Wisconsin and south to South Carolina, Georgia, Tennessee, Arkansas, and Missouri.

**What:** Harvest the roots.

**When:** Harvest roots in the fall when plant growth has stopped and the seed has matured. Harvest older more mature roots from the patch, leaving the younger ones for the future. Leave at least 20% of any patch you find to reseed. Rotate your patches from year to year.

**How:**  See Page 10-11 for general guidelines on cleaning, drying, and preparing roots for market.

Black Cohosh roots will dry whole, out of the sun. Be sure the root is thoroughly dry before storing. Store in paper or burlap bags. Never use plastic bags for storing roots.

**Cultivation:**  Black Cohosh likes a rich, moist, humus soil, and it likes humidity. It grows well in partial or filtered shade, and is best propagated by root division. Divide roots in the early spring or in the fall after plants are two years old. Root cuttings may take as long as two months to grow strong enough for transplanting. If starting from seeds, gather seeds in fall and keep moist. Start seeds in the fall for plants in the spring.

**Uses:**  Used by Native American women for menstrual and menopausal discomforts and for childbirth. Also used for nervous conditions, snakebite, high blood pressure, and arthritis. Black Cohosh is not recommended for use during pregnancy.

## <u>Notes</u>

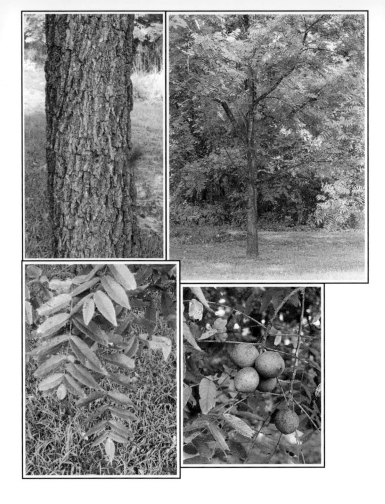

# Black Walnut
*Juglans nigra*

**Also Called:**   American Walnut, Eastern Black
Walnut, Walnut

**Description:**

Black Walnut is a valuable timber tree that averages 50 to 75 feet but can grow to 120 feet with a trunk clear of branches to 50 feet. When growing in the open without competition the limbs spread widely and form a majestic dome. When found in forests in competition with other trees, the crown is much narrower.

*Leaves:* Leaves grow from 12 to 24 inches long and are composed of 10 to 24 leaflets. The leaflets grow slightly alternate on a downy leaf stalk. They are shiny dark green, finely toothed, and their underside is slightly downy. Leaflets grow 3 to 3½ inches long, and the terminal leaflet is frequently under-developed or missing.

*Bark:* Black Walnut bark is dark brown to black, divided in rough ridges by narrow furrows, and has a diamond shaped pattern.

*Fruit:* The Black Walnut is round, growing 1½ to 2 inches in diameter with a thick, rough husk. The husk is furrowed and bright green early, turning dark brown to black as it dries and breaks open. The nut itself has a hard rough deeply furrowed shell, and the meat is oily and sweet.

**Where:** Black Walnut grows throughout the Eastern United States from the southern Great Lakes states east to southern Vermont and Massachusetts, south to Florida, Mississippi, and Louisiana, and west to Oklahoma, Texas, Kansas, and South Dakota. Black Walnut prefers the moist, rich well-drained soil of bottom lands and fertile hills. It grows tallest when in full sun.

**What:** Harvest bark, leaves, and fruit.

**When:** Harvest bark in the spring or early summer as the sap rises. Harvest leaves throughout the summer, and the fruit when mature.

**How:** See Page 10 for guidelines on harvesting barks, and Page 12 for cleaning, drying, and preparing for market. When harvesting leaves, take special care not to damage the tree or its branches. Black Walnut husks should be separated from the nuts and thoroughly dried before storing in paper or burlap bags.

**Uses:** Infusions from the leaves of Black Walnut have been used in treating ringworm, scabies, and other skin conditions. The bark is used as a mild laxative, and both green and dried hulls are effective in treating intestinal worms and other parasites. In some countries the juice of the fresh green hulls is used to treat hypothyroidism.

## <u>Notes</u>

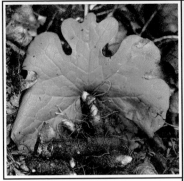

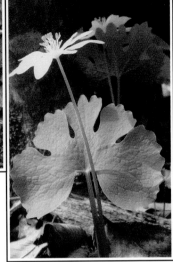

# Bloodroot
*Sanguinaria canadensis*

**Also Called:** Redroot, Red Indian Paint, Puccoon

**Description:** Bloodroot grows from 6 to 14 inches in height. Each plant has a single leaf and a single flower.

*Leaves:* Leaves are usually wrapped around the stem when the plant flowers and don't open fully until after the flower has bloomed. Leaves are a yellowish green and round-lobed, growing from 8 to 10 inches across.

*Flowers:* Bloodroot flowers are white, 1 to 2 inches across, and usually have 8 petals. The plant blooms from March to May, and the delicate

27

flowers last only a day or two.

*Roots:* Roots are generally small, from 1 to 4 inches in length and from ¼ to ½ inch thick, with many orange-colored rootlets. They are round and fleshy when freshly dug. When broken, they are a bright red on the inside and ooze a blood-red juice.

**Where:** Bloodroot grows in deep, cool, moist woods with rich soils. Often found growing with Solomon's Seal and May Apple. Grows from Quebec south to Florida and west to Texas and Kansas.

**What:** Harvest the roots.

**When:** Harvest in the late summer or fall when plant growth has stopped and the seed has matured. At this time the root has less moisture and is easier to dry. Many diggers mark their patches in the spring when the plant flowers and then dig in the late summer or fall. Harvest older, more mature roots from the patch, leaving the younger ones for the future. Leave at least 20% of any patch you harvest to reseed.

**How:** See Page 10-11 for general guidelines on cleaning, drying, and preparing roots for market.

Dirt is often caught in the root hairs of Bloodroot and needs to be removed by rinsing thoroughly and carefully. Because of their small size, these roots dry fairly quickly in a well ventilated area out of the sun.

Bloodroot tends to mold more easily than other roots. While they are drying, care should be taken to protect roots from the morning and evening dew. Roots must be thoroughly dry before storing. If bagged before dry, roots can mold, even if stored in paper or burlap bags. Do not store in plastic bags.

**Cultivation:** Bloodroot can be grown in shady areas where it receives protection from full sun. Plants can be grown from the seeds, which appear about 4 weeks after the flower blooms. For good germination, the seeds should be kept moist and planted immediately after gathering. Plant in loose, rich, well drained soil. Keep the beds moist, mulching with leaves, bark chips, or straw to help the soil retain moisture. If beds dry out, germination can be delayed by a year.

To establish by root division, dig in the late summer when the leaves have turned yellow. Cut the rhizome into pieces so that each piece has at least one bud. Plant immediately.

**Uses:**

Bloodroot is toxic and should be used with caution. Native Americans used the root to induce vomiting, treat fever, coughs, sore throat, bronchitis, and other lung ailments. Used today as a plaque inhibitor in mouthwash and toothpaste.

## Notes

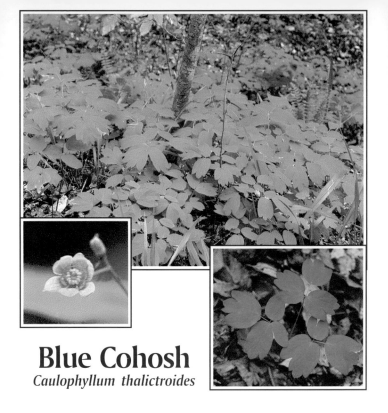

# Blue Cohosh
*Caulophyllum thalictroides*

**Also Called:** Blueberry, Blueberry Cohosh, Blue Ginseng

**Description:** In the early spring, Blue Cohosh sends up a bluish stem. This stem divides into 3 stems, and each of these stems divide into three.

*Leaves:* Each division produces 3 leaflets. These leaflets are oval in shape and have 3 to 5 lobes.

31

The stem and leaves of the newly emerging plant are covered with a bluish film.

*Flowers:* The small flowers are greenish yellow. They grow in clusters from the crook of the stem and bloom from April to June.

*Fruit:* The flowers are followed by blue seeds that resemble blueberries. These can be found on the plant in late August and into September.

*Roots:* The root is knotty and has small branches. The underside of the root has many long, matted rootlets.

**Where:** Blue Cohosh grows in deep, moist, rich woods. It ranges from New Brunswick to South Carolina and west to Nebraska.

**What:** Harvest the roots.

**When:** Dig Blue Cohosh root in the fall, after the seed has set. Seeds should be planted for future growth. Harvest older, more mature roots, leaving the younger ones to provide future harvests. Rotating patches from year to year is a sound harvesting practice.

**How:** See Page 10-11 for general guidelines on cleaning, drying, and preparing roots for market.

Roots need to be thoroughly cleaned. Rinse roots repeatedly in running water to loosen dirt that is caught in the hair roots. Rinse until water comes away clear. Roots should be dried whole, out of the sun.

**Uses:** Used by Native American women to induce menstrual flow, relieve cramps, and treat uterine inflammations. Also used for kidney and bladder infections, sore throat, and colic. Blue Cohosh is irritating to mucous membranes. Do not use during pregnancy.

## Notes

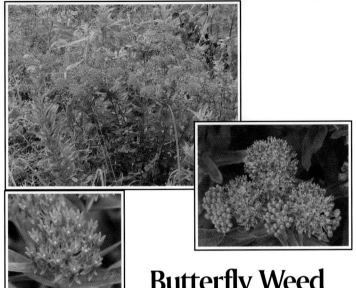

# Butterfly Weed

### *Asclepias tuberosa*

**Also Called:** Pleurisy Root, Chigger Weed, True Butterfly, Butterfly Milkweed

**Description:** A perennial plant that sends up several stems from each root cluster. The plant grows from 1 to 3 feet, branching at the top.

*Leaves:* The stems are covered with narrow leaves that are dark green on top and a pale green underneath. They grow alternately along the stems and are 2 to 6 inches long.

*Flowers:* Flowers are a brilliant, dark orange color, and grow in

35

showy clusters at the tops of the stems. Butterfly Weed flowers most of the summer and into the early fall.

*Seed Pods:* Butterfly Weed is a member of the milkweed family, and its flowers are followed by narrow seed pods measuring 4 to 5 inches. These pods contain the seeds with long, silky hairs like other milkweed plants.

*Roots:* The root consists of a long, branching tap root. It is white and fleshy when freshly dug. When dry, it wrinkles both lengthwise and across the root.

**Where:** Butterfly Weed grows in the open in dry, sandy, or rocky soil along the edges of forests, pastures, and roadsides. It can be found from Ontario to Minnesota, south to Florida, Texas, and Arizona.

**What:** Harvest the roots.

**When:** Dig Butterfly Weed root in the fall when plant growth has stopped and the seed pod has formed. Harvest older, more mature roots from the patch, leaving the younger ones for the future. Leave at least 10% of any patch you harvest to reseed.

**How:** See Page 10-11 for general guidelines on cleaning, drying, and preparing roots for market.

These large roots can be split to speed drying time. Never use an oven, microwave, wood stove, hot tin roof, or the back of your car to speed drying. When roots are thoroughly dry, store them in paper or burlap bags. Do not store in plastic bags.

**Cultivation:** Butterfly Weed is a hardy plant that grows well even in poor soil. Soil needs to be well drained, as rich soil that retains moisture will cause the roots to rot. Grows best in full sun, but will tolerate some shade.

Fresh seeds can be sown when a plant is collected. When sown in flats, seedlings need to be transplanted to larger pots when the second set of leaves appear. Plant in permanent beds as soon as the plants are established. If seedlings become pot-bound, they will deteriorate.

Plants can also be started from root cuttings in the fall. Cut the taproot into 2 inch pieces and place in rooting mixture outdoors in the shade.

Keep slightly moist. Mulch lightly with rotted leaves.

**Uses:** Used to treat all respiratory problems including bronchitis, pleurisy, pneumonia, and asthma. Also used to induce sweating to break up colds, fevers, and flu.

## Notes

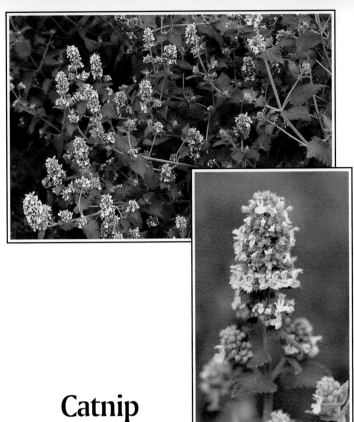

# Catnip
*Nepeta cataria*

**Also Called:**  Nip, Catmint, Catwort

**Description:**  This perennial plant grows upright and can reach 3 feet in height. The stems are square and branching.

*Leaves:* Leaves are opposite each other along the stems,

39

heart-shaped, and toothed. They are covered with tiny gray hairs that give Catnip a grayish-green look.

*Flowers:* Flowers are white or pale lavender with purplish spots. They are tube-shaped and grow in clusters at the ends of the main stem and the branches. Catnip flowers from June to September. The plant has a minty smell.

**Where:** Catnip can be found along roadsides, fence rows, stream banks, and other waste places throughout the United States. It can be easily cultivated.

**What:** Harvest the leaves, stems, and flowers.

**When:** Harvest Catnip when the plant is in bloom (June to September). Harvest on sunny days, late in the morning after the dew has dried. Do not pull on the plants, but cut them off above the ground, leaving the roots undisturbed. The roots will produce new plants the following season. Leave at least 10% of the patch to reseed.

**How:** See Pages 11-12 for general guidelines on cleaning, drying, and preparing herbs for market.

Be sure to dry out of the sun so the

plant material will retain its color and not turn brown. Protect from dew in the evenings and mornings. When thoroughly dry, store in paper or burlap bags. Do not store in plastic bags.

**Cultivation:** Easily started from seeds, either in pots or directly in the soil. Catnip likes an average to sandy, well-drained soil. Grows best in full sun, but will tolerate partial shade.

Catnip can be easily root divided after its second year of growth. Catnip also easily reseeds itself.

**Uses:** Used to treat colds and coughs, relieve chest congestion, and calm nervous conditions. Also used for infant colic, stomach cramping, and gas.

## Notes

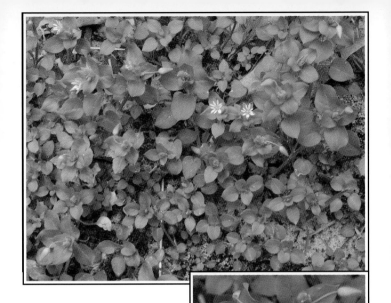

# Chickweed
*Stellaria media*

**Also Called:** Starweed, Star Chickweed, Stitchwort

**Description:** Chickweed is a low growing plant with weak straggling stems that branch freely. The plant can become invasive as its trailing stem will put down roots at the leaf junctions. In temperate climates it will remain green all winter.

*Leaves:* Leaves are opposite on the stem. They are small (½

43

inch), smooth, and oval with a point at the tip. In the evening the leaves fold over the growing tip to protect it.

*Stems:* The stems are juicy and pale green. A single line of fine hairs runs up the stem on one side only. This line of hairs changes sides as it reaches each leaf junction.

*Flowers:* Chickweed flowers continuously except in the dead of winter. The small ¼ inch flowers are 5-petaled, white, and each petal is deeply notched. They close in the evening and open in the morning.

**Where:** Chickweed is common throughout the United States and can be found in yards, fields, and around dwellings. It prefers moist, shady places and is at its best in early spring and fall when the weather is cool.

**What:** Harvest the entire above-ground part of this plant. It is best to cut the plant at the ground level, as the roots are shallow and fragile.

**When:** Chickweed is best harvested in early spring and summer.

**How:** See Pages 11-12 for general guidelines

on cleaning, drying, and preparing herbs for market.

Be sure to remove leaves, twigs, pine needles, and other foreign plant matter that may be entangled in the trailing stems and leaves.

**Uses:** Chickweed is full of vitamins and minerals and has been used as a green vegetable for centuries. Internally, Chickweed has been used to relieve coughs from congestion, asthma, and bronchitis. Externally Chickweed has been used to relieve various skin conditions including inflammations, ulcers, and itching. Chickweed is also said to be helpful in weight loss.

## Notes

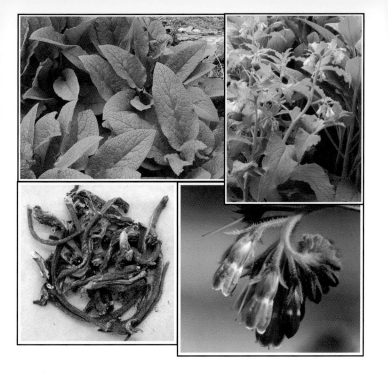

# Comfrey
*Symphytum officinale*

**Also Called:** Knitbone, Bruisewort, Healing Herb

**Description:** Comfrey is a coarse looking perennial plant with stout stems, large rough leaves, and large deep roots. Comfrey grows to 3 feet, dies back in the winter, and comes back vigorously every spring.

47

*Leaves:* Leaves are large, oval to lance-shaped, rough, and coarsely hairy.

*Flowers:* Comfrey flowers are bluish-purplish to white and tubular shaped. They bloom in clusters from May to July or August.

*Roots:* Comfrey roots are large, branched, and fleshy. They are wrinkled, brownish-black on the outside, and white inside.

**Where:** Comfrey is most often cultivated, although it has escaped from cultivation and grows in the wild. It grows best in rich soils, along stream banks, and in moist fields and meadows. There is also a Wild Comfrey (*Cynoglossum virginianum*) that grows mainly in Kentucky, Tennessee, and surrounding states.

**What:** Both the root and the above-ground part of the plant are harvested.

**When:** The above-ground part is best harvested at the time of flowering. The roots are best harvested in the fall, after the seed has set, and through to early spring before the new leaves appear.

**How:** See Pages 11-12 for general guidelines on cleaning, drying, and preparing herbs for market.

Comfrey leaf stalks and stems are very fleshy and subject to quick decay. It is best to strip the leaves from the stalk and dry them in single layers on screens in an area where you can keep air and a steady heat moving around them. When improperly dried the leaves will turn dark brown to black and can not appropriate for market or use.

See Pages 10-11 for general guidelines on cleaning, drying, and preparing roots.

**Cultivation:** Comfrey is remarkably easy to grow. It is easiest to start by root division in the fall, but can also be propagated by seed and cuttings. Plants should be set 3 feet apart. Comfrey grows best in moist rich soil and full sun to partial shade. Once established, Comfrey is a tough plant to get rid of, so care needs to be taken in choosing a location for growing. Once started, Comfrey grows very easily and requires little maintenance.

**Uses:** Comfrey has been used for centuries to promote healing of wounds, bruises, ulcers, and broken bones. Comfrey poultices have also been used for pulmonary problems including pneumonia and bronchitis.

Use of Comfrey roots internally is not recommended due to high levels of alkaloids that can cause liver damage.

### Notes

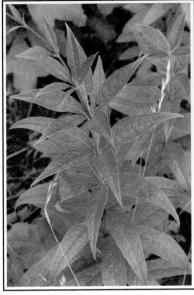
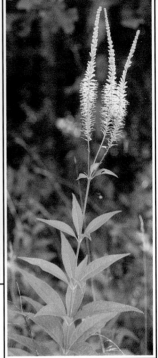

# Culver's Root
*Veronicastrum virginicum*

**Also Called:** Blackroot, Tall Speedwell, Culver's Physic, Leptandra

**Description:** Culver's Root is a perennial plant that grows straight up from the ground with no branches. It can reach from 2 to 6 feet in height.

*Leaves:* The leaves are found in whorls around the stem and each whorl is made up of 3 to 7

leaves. Leaves are narrow and lance-shaped. They grow from the base of the plant up the stem to the flower.

*Flowers:* The flowers grow at the top of the plant in showy spikes. They are small, white, and tube-like, blooming from June to September.

*Roots:* Roots grow from 4 to 6 inches in length. They are thick and branching with masses of small, brittle rootlets growing from the underside.

**Where:** Culver's Root grows in a variety of places, from dry or moist uplands to rich, moist woodlands and thickets, meadows, and prairies. It ranges from Massachusetts to Florida, west to Eastern Texas.

**What:** Harvest the roots.

**When:** Harvest Culver's Root from plants at least two years old. Harvest in the fall after plant growth has stopped and the seed has matured. Harvest older, more mature roots from the patch, leaving the younger ones for the future. Leave at least 25% of any patch you harvest to reseed. Mark your patches in the spring and summer for digging in the late fall and winter. Plants will return from the rootlets that are left after harvesting.

**How:**     See Pages 10-11 for general guidelines on cleaning, drying, and preparing roots for market.

Patience in allowing roots to dry thoroughly is important. If bagged before dry, even in paper or burlap, roots can mold. Never use an oven, microwave, wood stove, hot tin roof, or the back of your car to speed drying.

**Uses:**    Used by Native Americans to stimulate the liver and normalize the flow of bile. Also used as a laxative and to induce vomiting. **Use only dried root. Freshly dug Culver's Root is highly toxic.**

## Notes

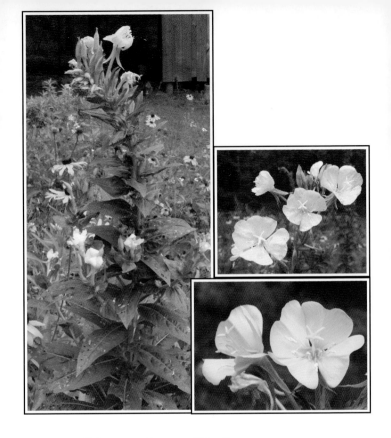

# Evening Primrose
### *Oenothera biennis*

**Also Called:**   Tree Primrose, Tall Sundrop

**Description:**   Evening Primrose is a biennial plant
that grows from 1 to 8 feet. It produces
a rosette of basal leaves and a
stalk the first year, and flowers

in the second year.

*Leaves:* Numerous lance-shaped, finely-toothed leaves grow alternately along the length of the stem. Leaves range from 2 to 6 inches in length.

*Flowers:* Yellow flowers bloom from early summer to early fall. The flowers have four wide petals and grow up to 2 inches across. Flowers open after sunset and close in the early morning. When closed, they look withered and limp and are an orangish-brown in color.

**Where:** Evening Primrose grows throughout the United States along roadsides, in waste places, and in dry open fields.

**What:** Harvest the entire above-ground part of the plant, including stem, leaves, and flowers.

**When:** Harvest Evening Primrose when it begins to flower. Harvest on sunny mornings after the dew has dried.

**How:** See Pages 11-12 for general guidelines on cleaning, drying, and preparing herbs for market.

Because Evening Primrose can grow up to 8 feet in height, it may be necessary to cut the plant into shorter lengths for drying. Air dry out of the sun on drying racks or cardboard flats, turning the plants occasionally to assure good air circulation. Protect from evening and morning dew. When thoroughly dry, store in paper or burlap bags.

**Uses:** Traditionally used in the treatment of asthmatic coughs and whooping cough. Evening Primrose has also been used externally to treat sores and various skin conditions. Oil extracted from the seeds has been shown to be useful for a number of conditions including eczema, asthma, inflammation, migraines, and PMS. The oil is a natural source of the essential fatty acid GLA.

## Notes

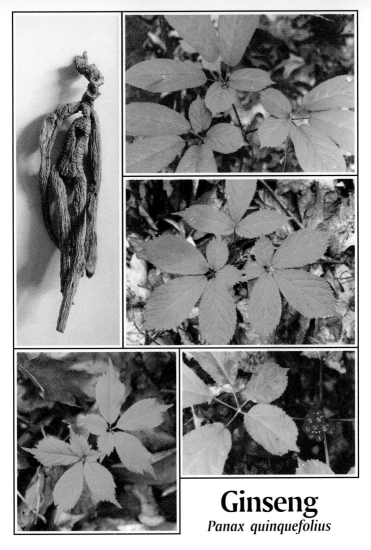

# Ginseng
*Panax quinquefolius*

**Also Called:** Sang, Manroot, Five-Fingers

**Description:** Ginseng is a perennial plant that grows up to 2 feet when

mature. The main stem produces three or more branches.

Each of these branches (or "prongs" as they are called by diggers) grows five leaves. Mature plants have three or more leaf stalks or prongs, with each stalk growing five leaves.

*Leaves:* The leaves all grow from the same point on the branch. Leaves are long and pointed on the ends, more rounded near the stalk, and the edges are toothed. The three outside leaves are larger than the two inside ones. In the late summer and early fall the leaves turn a golden yellow.

*Flowers:* The Ginseng flower grows where the leaf stalks come together on the main stem. The flowers are an unremarkable greenish yellow and bloom in June and July.

*Fruit:* The flowers are followed in the fall by bright red berries which carry the seeds.

*Roots:* Wild Ginseng roots range in size, depending on age and growing conditions. The immature roots are gener-ally small and simple. It is not until the root begins to mature that it becomes forked or branched. Roots from immature plants will be long and stringy, weigh less than older roots, and should be left to mature. Mature wild roots range from 3 to 8 inches in length and can be 2 to 3 inches thick. Freshly dug roots are prominently marked with wrinkles. They are pale yellow white to brownish white, and somewhat flexible. Properly cleaned and dried Ginseng roots are solid and firm, yellowish white in color with brownish wrinkles.

**Where:** Ginseng grows in deep, cool, hardwood forests. It grows best on land that slopes to the north or east, in areas that are shaded by a high canopy of trees. Although it is often found close to running water, it will rarely be found in damp places where water is standing or stagnant. Ginseng is often found growing in small communities. If you find one plant, you can generally find others in the same area.

**What:** Harvest the roots and tops.

**When:** The roots and tops of Ginseng are harvested in the fall, after the seeds have set. Check in your state for the legal Ginseng season. Harvest only the older, more mature plants from a patch, those with three or more prongs (leaflets). Leave the rest

61

to mature. Always plant seeds back in shallow soil to ensure future plants for the patch.

**How:**

See Pages 10-11 for general guidelines on cleaning, drying, and preparing roots and tops for market.

**Ginseng root should never be broken, split, or strung for drying.** The root needs to be whole and intact. Patience in drying is a must! Ginseng roots can take up to a month to dry properly. When dried slowly, the root dries from the inside out. As the inside dries and shrinks, it draws the skin, leaving it wrinkled.

**Never use an oven, microwave, wood stove, hot tin roof, or the back of your car to dry Ginseng.** Roots that are fast dried in this way form a hard, smooth shell on the outside. **Be sure your Ginseng is thoroughly dry before bagging it, and always store the roots in paper or burlap bags.**

Freshly dug roots lose weight on drying, depending on the time of year harvested and the amount of rainfall during that period. A 4 pound bag of wet roots dug earlier in the season can dry away to 1 pound. Later in the season shrinkage may be 3 pounds wet to 1 pound dry.

**For Our Grandchildren:** Dig Ginseng according to the state laws where you live. Most states specify that Ginseng should be dug after the fruits have ripened and the seed is ready for planting. After digging the roots, remember to replace the soil in the hole and plant the seeds in shallow soil. This will help insure future growth of the plant.

**Cultivation:** Ginseng is a difficult, expensive, and demanding plant to cultivate. A grower must be willing to commit several years of time and energy before harvesting the first crop. Plants require 70-80% shade, a rich, acidic soil, and a continuing supply of mulch. If grown in beds covered with lath and shade cloth, growers find it necessary to sterilize the soil to prevent mildew and fungal diseases, and to use herbicides to prevent weed growth. Prices paid for cultivated Ginseng are substantially lower than for wild dug.

Some diggers have successfully scattered Ginseng seeds in the woods and let nature take its course. Occasionally underbrush may need to be cut and removed, but the ground is not cultivated, nor the plants tended. Planted in the natural leaf mulch of the hardwood forest floor, the seeds are left alone to survive and grow. Areas that slope to the north and east, provide 80-90% shade, and have moist, rich, well-drained soil are best for this woods grown Ginseng. Some plants may be lost to moles and mice, but mildew and fungus, frequent problems in beds cultivated under lath, do little harm to plants in a more natural setting. Woods grown Ginseng sells for about half the price of Wild Ginseng, depending on the age and quality.

**Uses:** Used as a tonic, an aphrodisiac, and an appetite stimulant by the Chinese for thousands of years. Native Americans used Ginseng to treat colds, fevers, vomiting, and nervous disorders. Research shows it stimulates the immune system and increases energy levels.

## Notes

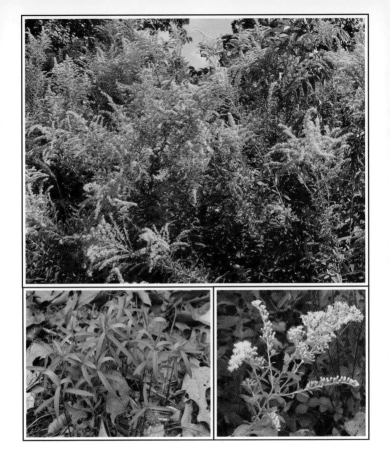

# Goldenrod
*Solidago odora, Solidago canadensis*

**Also Called:** *Odora:* Sweet Goldenrod, Anise Scented
Goldenrod, Blue Mountain Tea

*Canadensis:* Canada Goldenrod,
Field Goldenrod

**Description:** Goldenrod is a tall, erect perennial with a somewhat woody stem that branches at the top. Growing to 7 feet in height, very showy yellow flower clusters bloom along the top branches in late summer.

**Leaves:** *Canadensis:* Leaves grow in profusion alternately along the tall stems. They are lance-shaped and sharply toothed.

*Odora:* Leaves are similar in size and shape to *canadensis*, but are not toothed. Leaves are very fragrant, smelling like licorice or anise.

**Flowers:** In both species plumes of bright yellow flowers bloom in numerous clusters on the upper side of the arching branches. Flowers bloom from August to early fall. The flowers on *odora* have the same anise-like fragrance as the leaves.

**Where:** Goldenrod grows best in poor soils.

*Canadensis*: Most often found in fields and along roadsides. Frequently found growing in large patches. *Canadensis* ranges from Arkansas to North Carolina north into Canada.

*Odora*: *Odora* is found in dry open woods. Generally not found in large patches. It grows in all of the eastern and Midwestern states except for New England.

**What:** Harvest the entire above-ground part of the plant.

**When:** Harvest Goldenrod in late summer when it is in flower.

**How:** See Pages 11-12 for general guidelines on cleaning, drying, and preparing for market.

Care needs to be taken in drying Goldenrod. It should be spread out into a single layer on screens immediately after harvesting. If not given plenty of circulating air it will turn black and musty.

**Cultivation:** Goldenrod grows best in poor soil. In rich soil it tends to get leggy and the stem is unable to support the flowering heads. Goldenrod is easy to grow and can be started in flats for transplanting, directly sown into the ground, or transplanted from a friend's patch. Grows best in full sun.

**Uses:** Leaf and flower tea has been used for fevers, coughs, dysentery, diarrhea, and stomach cramps. Also used as a digestive stimulant. May cause allergic reactions in some people.

Notes

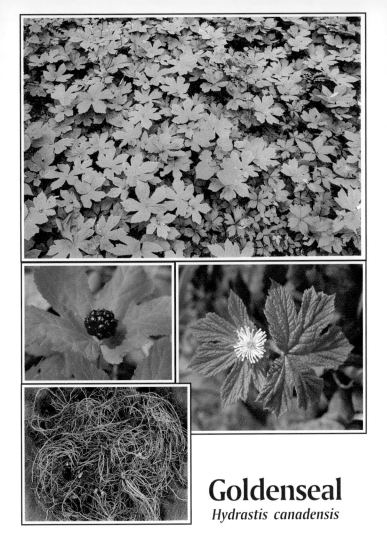

# Goldenseal
*Hydrastis canadensis*

**Also Called:** Yellow Root, Indian Paint, Yellow Puccoon

**Description:** Goldenseal grows from 6 to 12

inches tall. Each plant has one stem which forks at the top and bears two leaves, one of which is generally larger than the other.

*Leaves:* The leaves have 5 to 7 pointed lobes and look similar to maple leaves. They grow to 8 inches wide and are covered with a fine down. The edges are finely toothed.

*Flowers:* A single greenish-white flower appears from April to May.

*Fruit:* The fruit forms from the flower in the late summer and fall. It is similar to a raspberry in color and shape.

*Roots:* Roots are small, seldom more than 2 inches long with many rootlets attached. Freshly dug roots are a bright yellow and dry to a brownish yellow gold.

**Where:** Goldenseal grows in rich moist woodlands and can often be found growing with Ginseng, Solomon's Seal, and Bloodroot. Given the right growing conditions, Goldenseal will spread, forming large patches. Native to North America, the plant grows from Vermont south to Alabama and Georgia, west to Arkansas, and north to Minnesota.

| | |
|---|---|
| **What:** | Harvest the stems, leaves, and roots. |
| **When:** | Stems and leaves are collected just as the plant flowers. Goldenseal roots are harvested in the late summer and fall, after the berries have ripened and the seed has set. Dig the larger, more mature plants, and leave the smaller for future harvesting. |
| | It is wise to find two or three patches and rotate your harvesting from year to year. Leave any hair rootlets and broken roots in the ground. These will take hold and produce new plants. If mature patches of Goldenseal are not harvested in a 5 to 10 year period, the plants will begin to degenerate. |
| **How:** | See Pages 10-12 for general guidelines on cleaning, drying, and preparing roots and tops for market. |
| | The tops of Goldenseal should be cut from the root at ground level. Tops should be dried out of the sun to retain their green color. |
| | Clean roots thoroughly. Clumps of dirt, small stones, and organic matter become entwined in these roots. Rinse with lots of running water to loosen the dirt that clings to the root hairs. Rinse until water comes away |

clean. Spread in a single layer to dry.

**Cultivation:** Although not an easy plant to cultivate, Goldenseal can be grown in conditions that mimic those where it is found in the wild. This plant needs lots of shade, so growing in a wooded area or using shaded beds is necessary to filter out direct sunlight. Be sure that any shading structure built is high enough to provide for good air circulation. If preparing beds in a wooded area, clear out undergrowth and small trees. Raised beds may be needed if the ground is compact.

Soil should be rich in organic matter and toward the acid side of the pH scale. Goldenseal is a shallow-rooted plant that spreads by sending out root runners from the main rhizome. If the soil is not loose and light, the runners have difficulty spreading and establishing new plants.

Goldenseal is best propagated by root cuttings or root division. In the fall, dig the root and cut the rhizome into pieces at least ½ inch long. Some planters prefer that each piece has a bud or swelling, but plants will develop even from the small root hairs. Plant cut roots or root pieces in prepared soil about ½ to 1 inch deep. Mulch the beds with 3 or 4 inches of rotted leaves, bark, rotted saw dust, or straw. These materials will help the soil retain moisture and enrich it as they decompose.

Space roots at least one foot apart. As the plants develop, the rhizome will send out runners which will develop new plants and fill the bed. Root hairs may take a full year to send up a shoot. Root cuttings should send up a shoot the following spring, and begin sending out runners the first summer. It takes 3 to 4 years from the planting of root cuttings or root pieces to develop a crop of marketable roots. Harvest the largest plants, leaving the small ones and replanting any small roots to regenerate the bed. Wise growers harvest every 2 to 3 years.

**Uses:** Used to treat all inflammations of the mucous membranes. Also used as an antibiotic and antiseptic on cuts and open wounds, as a mouthwash, an eyewash, and an immune system stimulant.

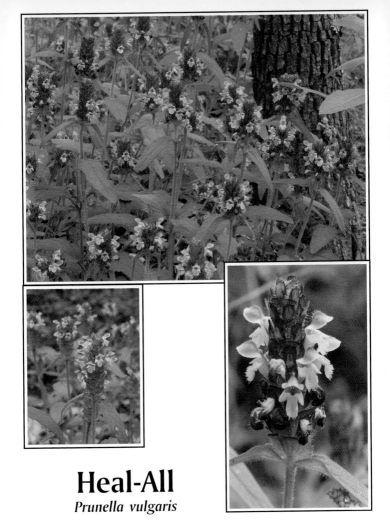

# Heal-All
*Prunella vulgaris*

**Also Called:** Self Heal, Carpenter's Herb

**Description:** Heal-All, an upright herbaceous perennial, is in the mint family.

It is referred to by many as a common weed and is often found in sprawling dense patches.

*Leaves:* Leaves are opposite and are oval to lance-shaped, although there may be a great deal of variation in leaf shape. Lower leaves have long stems while the upper ones are mostly stemless.

*Stems:* Heal-All stems are square as most mints are, and they are oftentimes hairy. The stem branches freely and grows to 12 inches in height.

*Flowers:* Flowers bloom in a cluster on a thickened, egg-shaped spike at the top of the stem. The flowers are two-lipped, with the upper lip hood-shaped and the lower one shorter and three-lobed. Flowers are lavender to white, and their nectar attracts bees and butterflies. Heal-All blooms from May to frost.

**Where:** Heal-All can be found throughout North America and is found in waste places, lawns, fence rows, and along roadsides.

**What:** Harvest the entire above-ground part of the plant including stem, leaves, and flowers.

**When:** Heal-All is best harvested as it begins to flower and throughout its blooming time.

**How:** See Pages 11-12 for general guidelines on cleaning, drying, and preparing herbs for market. Be sure the flower head is thoroughly dry before storing in paper or burlap bags.

**Uses:** Traditionally Heal-All has been used internally for sore throats, fevers, diarrhea, and as a diuretic. Externally, Heal-All has been used for wounds, bruises, boils, and ulcers. Recent research suggest Heal-All has antibiotic and anti-tumor properties.

## Notes

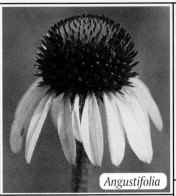

*Angustifolia*

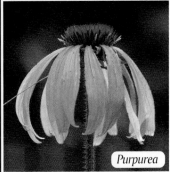

*Purpurea*

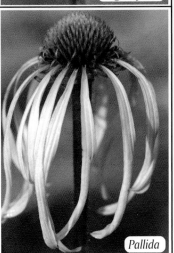

*Pallida*

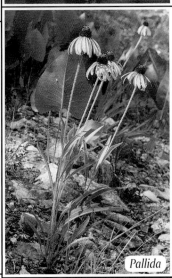

*Pallida*

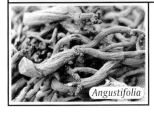

*Angustifolia*

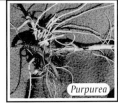

*Purpurea*

# Kansas Snake Root

*Echinacea angustifolia, pallida, purpurea*

79

**Also Called:** Echinacea, Purple Coneflower, Red Sunflower, Black Sampson

**Description:** These perennial plants grow from 6 inches to 3 feet tall on sturdy stems.

**Leaves:** *Angustifolia and Pallida:* Both of these species of Coneflower have narrow, oblong or lance-shaped leaves that grow from the bottom of the stem. Leaves and stem are thick and covered with bristly hairs.

*Purpurea:* This species has smaller, wider leaves than the other two. They are hairy and unevenly toothed and grow on the hairy stems.

**Flowers:** Flowers of these species are easily identifiable by their drooping petals.

*Angustifolia:* Flowers are smaller than the other two species, with the petals growing only an inch or two in length. Color ranges from pale pink to deep purple. Flowers bloom from June through late summer.

*Pallida:* Flowers have long drooping petals, sometimes growing as long as 4 to 5 inches. Petals are generally narrower than those of *Angustifolia* and range in color from purple to almost white. Cone heads vary in color from green to a rusty brown. Blooms from June through August.

*Purpurea:*  Petals are similar to *Angustifolia*, but longer with the color ranging from a deep pink-purple to white. Easily distinguished from the other two species by the bright orange cone head.

Roots:  *Angustifolia and Pallida:*  Both of these species have thick, long, taproots that twist lengthwise. Dried root is grayish brown on the outside and wrinkled lengthwise. The roots have a distinct, sweetish odor.

*Purpurea:*  Roots are more fibrous and there is no main tap root. Roots range from 2 to 3 inches long. The main root is knobby on top where the stem is and has many smaller roots growing off of it.

Where:  *Angustifolia:* Dry open places like prairies, open woods, and fields. Native range is the prairies of Western Kansas, Nebraska, Oklahoma, and North Dakota; west to Montana and Colorado; and north into Canada. Can be found growing in large stands.

*Pallida:*  Poor and rocky soils, glades, and roadsides. Ranges from Wisconsin and Minnesota south

81

to Texas and Arkansas, and west to eastern Kansas, Nebraska, and Oklahoma. Can be found growing in large stands.

*Purpurea:* Prefers a more moist soil than the other two species, and tolerates some shade. Often found growing alone or in small colonies in open woods near springs or where water seeps. It ranges throughout the central and southeastern United States, from Michigan and Ohio south to Louisiana, west to Texas and Oklahoma, and east to Georgia and Maryland.

**What:** Harvest the roots and flowering tops of all three species.

**When:** Harvest tops when plants are in bloom from June to end of July. Roots are harvested in the fall after the seed cone has ripened. Leave at least 10% of any patch to reseed for future harvesting. Pieces of taproot that are left in the ground will reproduce future plants. Appropriate harvesting of this plant helps maintain healthy stands. If it is not harvested, patches will become overcrowded and the plants will begin to deteriorate.

**How:** See Pages 10-12 for general guidelines

on cleaning, drying, and preparing roots and herbs for market.

Clean roots by rinsing with running water. Do not scrub. Even though some of these roots may be large, be patient and let them dry whole.

**Cultivation:** All species can be grown from seed. Collect seeds 4 to 6 weeks after flowering. When you bend the seed head over, seeds should fall out of the cone. Cut stems below the seed heads and drop into a paper bag. You will need to clean the seeds out from the chaff. Seeds can be directly sown after harvest or started in the early spring in flats for transplanting.

If planting in flats, the seeds need to be stratified. To stratify, place in moist sand and refrigerate. *Purpurea* needs to be stratified for at least 4 weeks. *Pallida* and *Angustifolia* need a 4-month period of stratification. Remove from refrigerator and put seeds into starting mix. These seeds need light to germinate, so do not cover them with soil. Place in a sunny window.

*Purpurea* germinates and develops fairly rapidly and can be planted in a permanent bed in 4 to 6 weeks.

Protect from the hot sun until well established. *Purpurea* may flower the first year if started early enough in the spring.

*Pallida* and *Angustifolia* are much slower to develop. Growth the first year may only reach 5 or 6 inches with few leaves. Flowers may not appear for two to three years.

*Angustifolia* prefers a more alkaline soil than the other two species. It is easily grown in its native territory (the prairies) but does not do well where summers are more humid.

Once established, these plants require very little in the way of care. They are generally hardy and very drought resistant. After a couple of years the patch will begin to reseed itself. It takes 3 to 4 years to establish roots for harvesting.

**Uses:** Used by the Native Americans for snakebite, spider bites, insect bites, boils, fevers, and blood poisoning. Echinacea is a nonspecific immune system stimulant that is currently used to treat colds, flu, and a host of other infections.

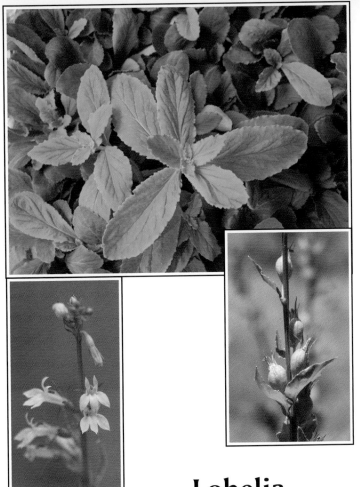

# Lobelia
*Lobelia inflata*

**Also Called:** Indian Tobacco, Bladder Pod, Puke
Weed, Emetic Weed, Asthma
Weed

**Description:** Lobelia is an annual or biennial herb growing 6 to 24 inches on hairy erect stems which contain a milky sap.

*Leaves:* Lobelia leaves vary from oval to oblong, are toothed and hairy on the undersides. Leaves are thin, light green and grow alternately. They measure 1 to 3 inches in length.

*Flowers:* Lobelia flowers are very small and inconspicuous. They have three oval petals facing downward and two sharply pointed petals facing up.

*Seed Pods:* As the flowers mature, the bottoms inflate to form seed capsules containing hundreds of tiny brown shiny seeds.

**Where:** Lobelia can be found in open woods, fields, waste places, and pastures. Lobelia grows from New England west to Minnesota and south from Arkansas through Mississippi, Alabama, and Georgia.

**What:** Harvest the entire above-ground part of the plant, including stems, leaves, and seed pods.

**When:** Harvest Lobelia when seed pods have matured. Leave at least 25% of any patch to reseed.

**How:** See Pages 11-12 for general guidelines on cleaning, drying, and preparing herbs for market. Dry Lobelia on a fine mesh screen with clean paper or cloth underneath to catch any of the tiny seeds that may fall through.

**Cultivation:** Lobelia can be sown outdoors in the spring or fall, or it can also be sown in flats or fine soil in January or early February. Seeds are small, and it is best to mix them with sand to keep seedlings separate from each other. Average germination time is 1 to 3 weeks in warm soils. Seedlings should be transplanted from flats to pots when they are large enough to handle and then set out in early June. Lobelia prefers part to full sun, rich moist soil and generous amounts of water.

**Uses:** Traditionally Lobelia leaves have been smoked to relieve asthma, bronchitis, sore throats, and cough. Also the plant has been widely used to induce vomiting and sweating and for its sedative and muscle relaxing properties. Lobelia is used in many quit smoking herbal and homeopathic preparations.

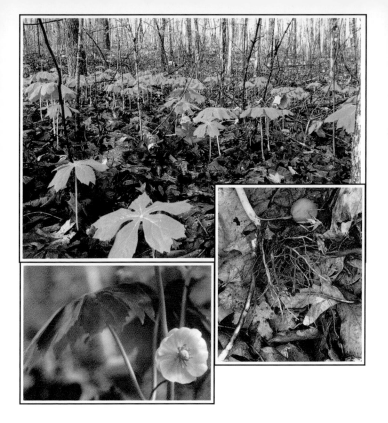

# Mayapple
*Podophyllum peltatum*

**Also Called:** Devil's Apple, Mandrake, Umbrella Plant, Indian Apple

**Description:** Often found growing in large patches, this early spring perennial grows 12 to 18 inches high.

*Leaves:*  Mayapple has a single stalk that often forks with two umbrella-like leaves at the top. Leaves are smooth, shiny, and large.

*Flowers:*  At the fork of the stem, a single white, waxy-looking flower blooms from April to June. The flower averages 2 inches across and matures into a plum-size yellow fruit. In any patch of Mayapple one can find a number of plants which bear no flowers or fruit.

*Roots:*  The root runs horizontally under the ground and can grow to 6 feet or longer. It is smooth and round and very flexible when freshly dug. On the upper surface of the roots are thickened scars of earlier stems and on the lower side, thick, stout masses of rootlets.

**Where:**  Mayapple grows best in rich, damp, open woodlands, near streams, in partial shade. It can also be found in open glades and clearings. Generally it is found growing in large patches, ranging from New England to Minnesota and south to Florida and Texas.

**What:**  Harvest the roots.

**When:**  Harvest roots in the late summer when plant growth has stopped, the leaves have yellowed, and the seed has matured. Harvest older, more mature roots from the patch, leaving the younger ones for the future. Remember when digging that mature Mayapple roots can grow six feet long or longer.

Leave at least 10% of any patch you find to reseed. Plants will also mature from rootlets left in the ground.

**How:**   See Pages 10-11 for general guidelines on cleaning, drying, and preparing roots for market.

Although these roots may be long, they are not often very thick and can be dried whole. Store only in paper or burlap bags and only when roots are thoroughly dry.

**Uses:**   Traditionally used as a regulator for liver and bowel functions, jaundice, and other liver ailments. Also used to remove warts. Potentially toxic. Large doses can cause nausea, vomiting, and intestinal inflammation.

## Notes

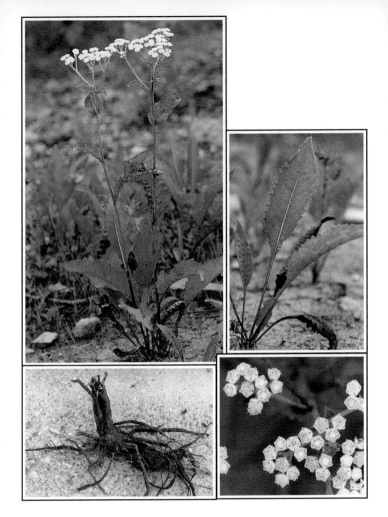

# Missouri Snakeroot
*Parthenium integrifolium*

**Also Called:** Wild Quinine, American Fever-few

**Description:** This perennial has stout stems that can grow to 5 feet and are topped with small white flowers.

*Leaves:* Leaves growing at the base of the stem are large and lance-shaped and can reach 1 foot in length. Smaller leaves grow alternately along the stem. Leaves are rough and hairy.

*Flowers:* Flowers appear from May to July. Each white flower is ¼ inch wide and many flowers cluster together, forming a flat-topped, umbrella-shaped mass.

*Roots:* The rootstock is large, thick, dark brown to black in color, with many smaller roots growing on the underside.

**Where:** Missouri Snakeroot grows in dry areas of prairies and open woods over much of the Eastern United States.

**What:** Harvest the roots.

**When:** Roots are harvested in the fall after the plant has gone to seed. It is wise to sow seeds from this plant, as it reproduces well and will insure future harvesting.

**How:** See Pages 10-11 for general guidelines on cleaning, drying, and preparing roots for market.

This plant is sometimes found growing in heavy, clay-type soil, making cleaning a chore. The roots are often tangled with clumps of dirt and small gravel. Running a hose over the roots will help loosen the dirt. Rinse until water comes away clear. Do not scrub. Large rootstock can be split to speed drying.

**Uses:**     Used for fevers, flu, as a diuretic, and for kidney and bladder problems.

## Notes

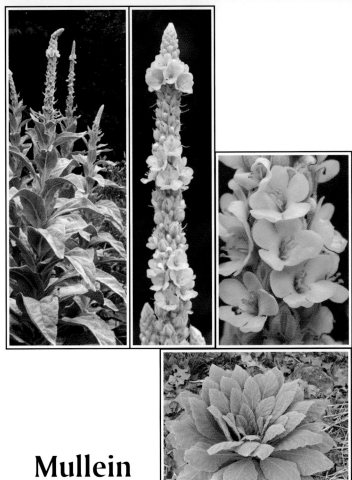

# Mullein
*Verbascum thapus*

**Also Called:** Common Mullein, Wooly Mullein,
Aaron's Rod, Flannel Leaf,
Indian Tobacco

97

**Description:** Mullein is a common roadside plant. It is a biennial plant, one that takes two years to flower and set seed. The first year a rosette of large downy leaves appear and the second year a tall conspicuous flowering stalk.

*Leaves:* Mullein leaves are thick, fuzzy, and felt-like. They are light sage-green and can grow more than a foot in length. During the first year the leaves form a rosette that can spread to 2 feet in diameter. The leaves are broad and oval or lance shaped. The leaves on the flower stalk are smaller and are alternate.

*Flowers:* The second year the Mullein plant sends up stout flower stalks that will sometimes branch. Stalks grow from 2 to 10 feet or better. The flower appear tightly packed around the stalk and bloom a few at a time from June to August. The flowers are yellow and small, growing an inch or less across. They have 5 petals that are fused together at the base and are cup shaped. The flower stalks are remarkably sturdy and stay erect through the winter if undisturbed.

**Where:** Mullein grows in dry fields and meadows, along roadsides and railroad tracks, in vacant lots, disturbed areas, and in open forests. It ranges throughout the United States.

**What:** Leaves, flowers, and roots are harvested.

**When:** Flowers can be harvested every other day or so throughout the summer. Leaves are harvested from both the first year's rosette and along the stalk before the flowers bloom. Roots are best harvested after flowering when the seeds have set.

**How:** See Pages 11-12 for general guidelines for cleaning, drying, and preparing herbs for market.

Be sure to allow sufficient time for the thick Mullein leaves to dry before storing them in paper or burlap bags.

Special care should be taken in drying the flowers. Spread them in on layer, out of the sun, with good ventilation.

**Uses:** Mullein leaves, flowers, and roots have been used to treat all manner of respiratory ailments including colds, sore throats, coughs, bronchitis, and asthma. Leaves have been used in teas, tinctures, and also smoked or smudged and the smoke inhaled to dilate the bronchioles, alleviate chest congestion, and expel mucus.

Mullein flowers, soaked in olive or mineral oil, have been used as earache drops.

### Notes

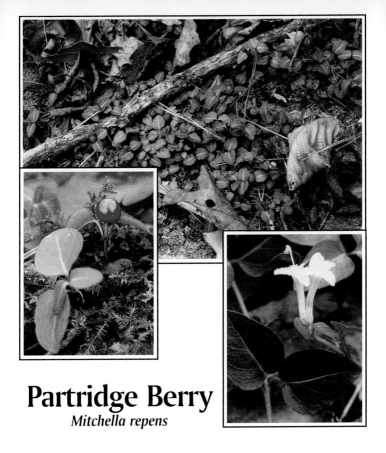

# Partridge Berry
*Mitchella repens*

**Also Called:** Squaw Berry, Squaw Vine, Winter Clover, Two-Eyed Berry, Hi-Vine

**Description:** Partridge Berry is a perennial evergreen vine that grows at the foot of forest trees and around decayed stumps. It can also be found growing along rock bluffs. Individual vines grow from 6 to 36 inches long. Often **101**

times many of these vines will be found growing together in a mass, making it difficult to tell where one vine stops and another begins.

*Leaves:* Leaves are small and grow opposite each other on either side of the stems. The top of the leaves are shiny green, and some have prominent white veins.

*Flowers:* Flowers are small (¼ inch wide), white, and funnel-shaped. They bloom from May to July and are found in pairs at the end of the vines.

*Fruit:* The two flowers merge to form a bright, scarlet-red berry. These berries stay red throughout the fall and winter, and if they are not eaten by birds, will often be found on the plant when the new flowers begin to bloom the following spring.

**Where:** Partridge Berry grows in shaded woods. It most frequently grows where it is moist and can often be found on rocky hillsides and bluff faces that seep water during the spring and fall. It grows from Eastern Canada to Minnesota, south to Texas, and east to Florida.

**What:** Harvest the entire above-ground part of the plant, including stems, leaves, and berries.

**When:** Harvest Partridge Berry from summer to fall. Harvest on sunny days, late in the morning after the dew has dried.

This vine will return year after year from the root if care is taken not to disturb the roots while harvesting the tops. Pulling on the plant can injure the shallow root system. It is best to cut the plant off above the ground. Leave at least 25% of the patch to reseed.

**How:** See Pages 11-12 for general guidelines on cleaning, drying, and preparing herbs for market.

Pick through Partridge Berry carefully to remove twigs, stones, and moss that get entangled with this vine when harvesting.

If drying outdoors, protect from dew in the evenings and mornings. When thoroughly dry, store in paper or burlap bags. Do not store in plastic bags.

**Uses:** Used by Native American women during pregnancy to aid in childbirth, for irregular or delayed menses, as a uterine tonic, and for sore nipples. Is also used for insomnia and as a diuretic.

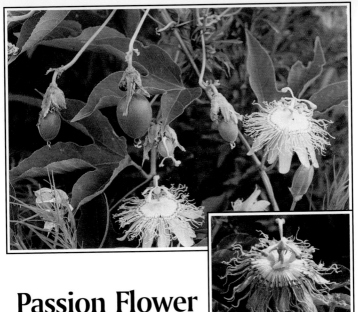

# Passion Flower
*Passiflora incarnata*

**Also Called:** Maypop, Apricot Vine

**Description:** Passion Flower is a climbing vine that can grow upwards to 30 feet.

*Leaves:* Its leaves grow alternately along the stem. They are a shiny green and have three long lobes that each come to a point. Their edges are very finely toothed. Long coiling tendrils grow from the underside of the stems, attaching the plant to any available support.

105

*Flowers:* Flowers are 1 to 2 inches across and unusually beautiful. Their petals are very narrow and radiate out from the center of the flower. They range in color from white to various shades of purple.

*Fruit:* The fruit grows from 2 to 3 inches and is round to oblong. Fruits are green when they form and ripen to a golden yellow. The fruit has an unusual, faintly tropical flavor and is filled with small seeds.

**Where:** Passion Flower grows along fence rows, in pastures, at the edges of wooded areas, and in partially shaded, dry areas, or thickets over much of the Midwest and South, ranging west into Texas and Oklahoma to the west. Many farmers find this plant to be a nuisance and might very well accept your offers to harvest it.

**What:** Harvest the entire above-ground part of this plant, including leaves, flowering tops, fruit, and stems.

**When:** Harvest Passion Flower when it begins to flower, from June to September. Frequently you will find both flower and fruit on the vine at the same time. Harvest on sunny days, late in the morning after the dew has dried. Passion Flower is a very sturdy vine and will return year after year as long as the roots aren't disturbed. Leave at least 10% of the patch to reseed. If harvesting from the wild, try not to harvest from the same patch year after year. Rotating among patches allows for reseeding and abundant regrowth.

**How:** See Pages 11-12 for general guidelines on cleaning, drying, and preparing herbs for market.

Because Passion Flower is a vine, twigs and leaves from other plants get caught into it when harvesting. Be sure to remove all foreign matter that may become entangled with the plant. Air dry out of the sun on drying racks or cardboard flats, turning the plants occasionally. Protect from dew in the evenings and mornings. When thoroughly dry, store in paper or burlap bags. Do not store in plastic bags.

**Cultivation:** Passion Flower is difficult to start from seed. Take stem cuttings in early spring and root in well-drained rooting medium. Protect from direct sunlight. Once established in the ground, numerous suckers will begin to appear. These can be dug and transplanted. Prefers a sandy soil. If soil is too rich, the plant will produce fewer flowers. Once started, Passion Flower spreads abundantly.

**Uses:**   Used by the Native Americans to treat bruises, burns, and skin problems. Also used for insomnia, restlessness, irritability, and other nervous conditions.

## <u>Notes</u>

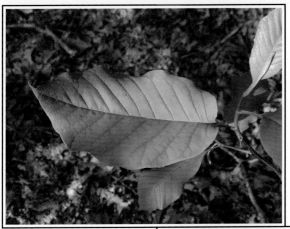

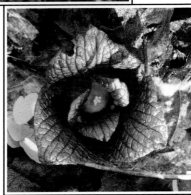

# Paw Paw
*Asimina triloba*

**Also Called:** Wild Banana, Custard Apple, Fetid Shrub

**Description:** Paw Paw is a small tree growing from 9 to 30 feet tall. The trunk is straight with thin gray bark marked by ash-colored blotches. Limbs are long, straight, and brittle. Paw Paw is generally an understory tree but can also be found growing in dense thickets.

*Leaves:* Paw Paw leaves are among the largest in the woods. Growing up to a foot in length, they are 4 to 6 inches broad, light green on top and paler underneath. Leaves emit a foul odor when bruised.

*Flowers:* Paw Paw flowers appear before the leaves. They begin as pale green and turn a dull, dark maroon. Flowers tend to droop with their petals curved backwards. Paw Paw blooms from March to May.

*Fruit:* Fruits are oblong, slightly curved, stubby, and grow 3 to 5 inches long. They are green at first and ripen to a brown. The flesh has a custard-like texture. Fruits ripen from July to September.

**Where:**  Paw Paw grows in rich soils, along stream banks, and in rich woods. It ranges from northern Florida to western New York state east to east Texas and southern Iowa.

**What:**  Harvest the twigs.

**When:** Harvest Paw Paw twigs in April and May.

**How:** Harvest the twigs using pruning shears. Harvest twigs no larger than ½ inch in diameter. Dry on screens out of the sun.

**Uses:** Paw Paw leaves have traditionally been used as a diuretic and as an insecticide. Recent research has found the leaves and twigs to contain anti-cancer properties.

## <u>Notes</u>

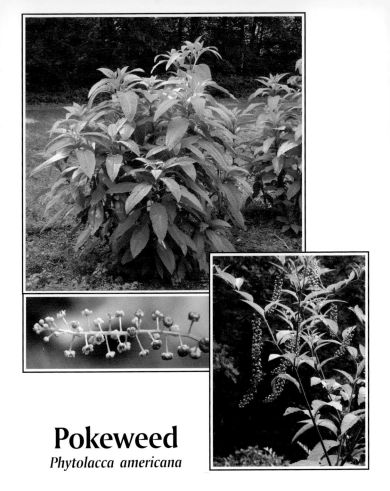

# Pokeweed
*Phytolacca americana*

**Also Called:** Poke, Pokeberry, Poke Sallet, Inkberry, American Nightshade, Cancer Root, Pigeonberry

**Description:** Pokeweed is a large rooted showy perennial plant with a

113

sturdy smooth purple stem
reaching to 10 feet or more.

*Leaves:* Leaves are alternate or scattered on the stem, large, toothless, and oval to oblong. They are a rich green, turning to yellow in the fall.

*Flowers:* An abundance of small greenish-white flowers bloom on plume-like racemes from mid-summer to early fall. Flowers seldom grow over ¼ inch and are borne on reddish stems.

*Fruit:* The flowers are followed by shiny green berries in grape-like clusters which mature to a smooth, shiny, deep purple. The berries are globular and flattened at both ends. Berries contain a crimson juice and small black seeds.

*Roots:* Pokeweed has a large, fleshy, branched root. The root is fibrous, whitish within, and covered with a thin brownish bark. It is easily cut or broken.

**Where:** Pokeweed grows abundantly anywhere in its range where the soil has been disturbed. It can be found along fencerows, in fields, waste places, and even on bulldozed piles of dirt and trees. It ranges from the New England states west to Minnesota and south to

Texas and Florida.

**What:**     Harvest roots, leaves, tender shoots.

**When:**     Harvest roots in the fall after berries have ripened and the plant begins to die back.

Harvest tender young shoots in the early spring for "poke sallet" or cooked greens.

**How:**     See Pages 10-11 for general guidelines on cleaning, drying, and preparing roots for market. Poke roots can be cut crosswise or lengthwise to speed drying.

When harvesting young shoots, be sure to cut above ground to avoid including any of the root.

**Uses:**     Pokeweed should be used with caution. All parts of the plant contain toxic substances, with more present in the roots and the red outer skin of the mature stalk. When used in high doses, Pokeweed acts as a purgative and emetic. It can also cause dermatitis.

All parts of the Pokeweed plant have been used for centuries to treat various conditions. The juice from the berries has been used to treat skin conditions. The root has been used in small doses as a blood cleanser, and for joint pain, breast tumors, and lymphatic swelling.

When preparing cooked greens, be sure to boil them twice, discarding the first water.

## Notes

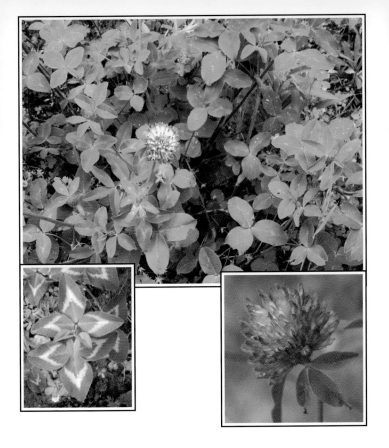

# Red Clover
### *Trifolium pretense*

**Also Called:** Sweet Clover, Purple Clover, Honeysuckle, Trefoil

**Description:** Red Clover is a short lived perennial or biennial with several stems arising from the same root.

117

Stems are hairy and vary in height from 18 to 26 inches.

*Leaves:* Leaves are divided into 3 leaflets that grow on alternate sides of the stem. The leaflets are broad, oval, and pointed. A white V-shaped pattern can be found near the middle of each leaf. The two top leaves are usually found close to the flower head.

*Flowers:* Flowers are found in tight, rounded heads measuring up to an inch wide. Each head consists of between 50 to 500 florets. Flowers range in color from pink to red to light purple and are fragrant. Red Clover blooms in late spring and continues to early fall.

**Where:** Red Clover can be found throughout the United States. It grows in a wide variety of environments including fields, roadsides, riverbanks, vacant lots, and open forests. It prefers well-drained loamy soil.

**What:** Harvest the entire above-ground part of the plant including stems, leaves, and flowers.

**When:** Harvest Red Clover in the summer when in full bloom.

**How:** See Pages 11-12 for general guidelines

on cleaning, drying, and preparing herbs for market. Take special care to keep out of the sun while drying to preserve the color of the flower heads. Flower heads turn brown when dried improperly.

**Uses:** Traditionally used as an antispasmodic, mild sedative, blood purifier, and for various lung problems including spasmodic coughs, asthma, and bronchitis. Red Clover has also been used extensively by many as a cancer remedy. Although modern science has failed to confirm the traditional uses of Red Clover, they do admit that it contains many biologically active compounds, one of which is being investigated for its possible anti-tumor activity.

### Notes

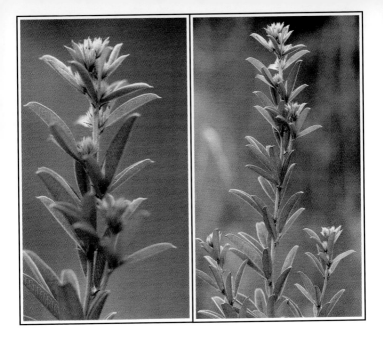

# Round-Headed Lespedeza
*Lespedeza capitata*

**Also Called:** Prairie Clover, Lespedeza, Bush Clover

**Description:** Round-Headed Lespedeza is a tall growing clover reaching between 2 and 5 feet in height. Very fine, silvery hairs cover the leaves and stems.

*Leaves:* The leaves grow alternately along the stem and resemble clover leaves with three leaflets.

*Flowers:* The flowers grow 121

close to the stem, mostly at the top of the plant. They are ½ to 1½ inches in diameter and a creamy white color. The plant gets the name "Round-Headed" from the shape of the flowers, which appear in closely packed clusters with round-shaped heads. Round-Headed Lespedeza blooms from July to September.

**Where:** Dry fields and prairies, open woodlands from New England west to Minnesota, south to Florida, and west to Texas.

**What:** Harvest the leaves, stems, and flowers.

**When:** Harvest the leaves, stems, and flowers when the plant is in bloom, July to September. Harvest on sunny days, late in the morning after the dew has dried. Do not pull on the plants, but cut them off above the ground and leave the roots undisturbed. The roots will produce new plants the following season. Leave at least 25% of the patch to reseed. Be aware that some areas where this Lespedeza grows may be subject to spraying with herbicides. Harvest only healthy, strong plants. Stunted or dried, brownish looking plants may indicate that the plants have been sprayed, and these plants should not be harvested.

**How:** See Pages 11-12 for general guidelines on cleaning, drying, and preparing herbs for market.

Be sure to store in paper or burlap bags. Plastic can cause the plant material to mold, scald, and turn black. When this happens, your crop has no medicinal or monetary value.

**Uses:** Traditionally used by Native Americans to treat rheumatism and neuralgia. Recent scientific studies show it may lower cholesterol levels and possess some anti-tumor activity.

## Notes

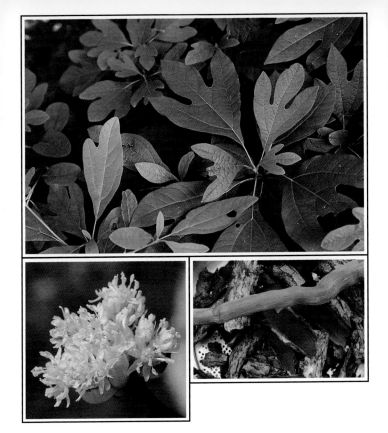

# Sassafras
## *Sassafras albidum*

**Also Called:** Cinnamon Wood, Smelling Stick, Ague Tree

**Description:** The Sassafras Tree grows from 10 to 40 feet in height. In the North it is more shrub-like, while in the

125

South it has been found growing up to 100 feet. The bark is rough, deeply channeled, and gray in color.

*Leaves:* Sassafras is easily identifiable by its leaves, which grow in three different mitten-shapes, having one, two, or no "thumbs." Leaves are 4 to 6 inches long and shiny green. Newly emerging leaves have a spicy smell and taste. Leaves turn yellow, orange, pink, and dark red in late summer.

*Flowers:* Clusters of small yellow flowers bloom from April to May, before the leaves appear.

*Roots:* The roots are thick and send up many suckers, often forming thickets. Older roots are large, woody, and have a reddish or grayish brown color. The root bark has a rough texture. The roots and root bark smell like root beer.

**Where:** Sassafras can be found along roadsides, in thickets, and in abandoned fields, as well as in the woods. It ranges from New England south to Florida and west to Texas.

**What:** Harvest leaves, root bark, and tree bark.

**When:** Sassafras leaves are harvested during

the growing season, root bark in late winter or early spring, and tree bark when the sap is rising in the spring and early summer.

**How:** See Pages 11-12 for general guidelines on cleaning, drying, and preparing barks and leaves for market.

Be sure to keep root bark and tree bark separate. The root bark stops at the top of the soil. Above that point is tree bark.

Tree bark is best gathered from the branches of the trees rather than the trunk. Never girdle the trunk or branches of the tree. Strip the bark from one side of branches only.

When thoroughly dry, be sure to bag bark in paper or burlap. Do not use plastic bags. Even the smallest amount of moisture will cause the bark to mold when stored in plastic.

**Uses:** Traditionally Sassafras has been used as a spring tonic to stimulate and cleanse the liver and purify the blood. Also used for stomachache, colds, and fever. Sassafras leaves are used in filé gumbo.

Notes

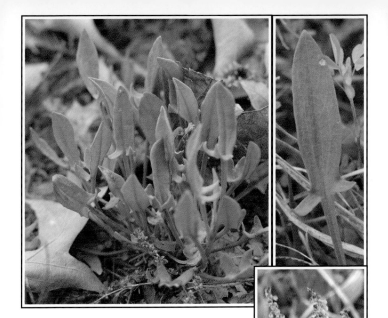

# Sheep Sorrel
*Rumex acetosella*

**Also Called:** Field Sorrel

**Description:** Sheep Sorrel is a perennial herb with a pleasantly sour tasting leaf. It is a slender plant and can be identified by the reddish tinge at the base of the leaves and the red seed head that forms after blooming.

129

*Leaves:* Leaves are arrow-shaped, slender, and vary from ½ to 2 inches in length. They have a sour, acid taste.

*Stems:* Multiple stems arise from the base of the plant growing from 3 to 4 inches to a foot tall. The stem branches at the top.

*Flowers:* Tiny flowers bloom along the branched upper stems from June to October. The flowers are green with a red tinge, turning a deep red-brown later in the summer as seed develops. Like Yellow Dock, this seed stalk stays on the plant throughout the winter.

**Where:** Sheep Sorrel is found throughout the United States. It is abundant in sandy, acidic, thin soils.

**What:** Harvest the entire above-ground part of the plant.

**When:** Harvest Sheep Sorrel as it begins to flower in early summer. Harvest on sunny days in late morning after the dew has dried.

**How:** See Pages 11-12 for general guidelines on cleaning, drying, and preparing herbs for market. Be sure to dry out of the sun to retain good color.

**Uses:** Sheep Sorrel is probably best known as one of the herbs in the Essiac Tea formula that has been used as a cancer remedy. Sheep Sorrel is also eaten as a spring green either cooked with other greens or added to salads.

### <u>Notes</u>

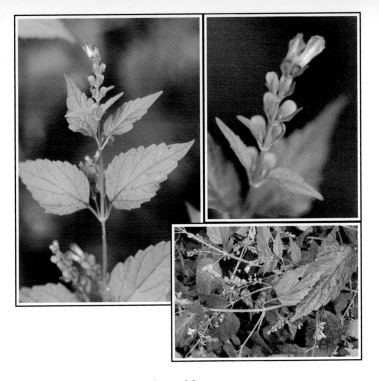

# Skullcap
*Scutellaria laterifloria*

**Also Called:** Mad Dog Skullcap, Sideflowering Skullcap, Quaker Bonnet, Helmet Flower

**Description:** Skullcap is an upright widely branching perennial that grows to three feet tall. The stem is slender and square.

*Leaves:* Leaves are 1 to 4 inches long, and grow opposite each other along the stems. They are wider at the stem end and come to a point at the tip. The edges are coarsely toothed.

*Flowers:* Flowers are small and range from a light violet to blue in color. They are tube-shaped and have two lips, the upper one hooded. The flowers grow on one side of spikes that grow from the crook of the leaves and stem. This placement of the flowers makes it easy to tell this medicinal plant from other non-medicinal Skullcaps whose flowers grow either in spikes at the top of the plant or singly at the junction between the leaves and stem. Skullcap flowers from June to September.

**Where:** Skullcap grows in moist, rich woods, along streams, and in or around swampy areas throughout the United States.

**What:** Harvest the leaves, stems, and flowers.

**When:** Harvest when the plant is in bloom, June to September. Harvest on sunny days, late in the morning after the dew has dried. Do not pull on the plants, but cut them off above the ground and leave the roots undisturbed. The roots will produce new plants the following season. Leave at least 10% of the patch to reseed. Try not to harvest from the same patch year after year. Rotating among patches allows for reseeding and abundant regrowth.

**How:**     See Pages 11-12 for general guidelines on cleaning, drying, and preparing herbs for market.

Be sure to pick through plant material to remove all foreign matter that may be entangled with the plant. If drying outside, protect from dew in the evenings and mornings. When the plant material is thoroughly dry, store in paper or burlap bags. Do not store in plastic bags.

**Uses:**     Skullcap was believed by some to cure rabies, giving rise the common name "Mad Dog Skullcap." This plant is an effective sedative and nervous system tonic. It is also used as a digestive aid.

## Notes

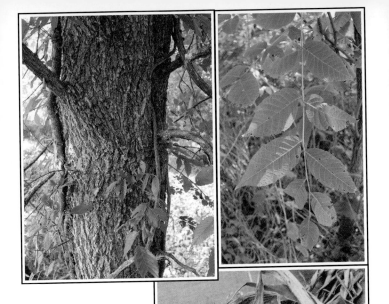

# Slippery Elm
### *Ulmus rubra*

**Also Called:**  Red Elm, Indian Elm, Sweet Elm, Soft Elm

**Description:**  Slippery Elm trees average from 40 to 60 feet in height, but can reach upwards to 100 feet in rich moist soils. The trunk rises free of branches for great heights, and its branches are erect and less drooping than its more well known cousin the American Elm.

**Leaves:** Slippery Elm leaves are 4 to 7 inches long and 2 to 3 inches wide with sharply double serrated edges. The base of the leaf is noticeably unequal. Leaves are thick dark green with very rough, stiff hairs on the upper surface and a soft hairy underside.

**Flowers:** Inconspicuous flowers appear early in the spring before the leaves open. The seeds ripen from April to June and are surrounded by a thin, circular, veiny, hairless wing.

**Bark:** The bark is thick with shallow fissures and raised, braided ridges. The inner bark is white, fragrant (some say it smells like maple syrup), and when chewed becomes mucilaginous or slippery.

**Where:** Slippery Elm grows best in moist rich soils of lower slopes and flood plains, but also grows on dry hillsides with limestone soils. It ranges from southern Quebec west to North Dakota, south to south-central Texas, and Florida.

| | |
|---|---|
| **What:** | Harvest bark, either natural (both inner and outer) or rossed (inner bark only). The inner bark is the white, chewy substance between the outer bark and the wood. |
| **When:** | Harvest bark in the spring (March to April) when the sap begins to rise. |
| **How:** | See Page 10 for general guidelines on harvesting barks. Bark should be stripped from only one side of branches or trunk. The tree will heal over where harvested and continue to grow. Never girdle the trunk or branches as this will kill the tree. For rossed bark, cut away the thick outer bark. |
| **Uses:** | Slippery Elm is highly nutritious and can be made into a broth for people debilitated by illness. Traditionally used for a number of gastrointestinal problems including stomach irritation, ulcers, diarrhea, and dysentery. Also used for sore throats, cough, and pleurisy. |

### Notes

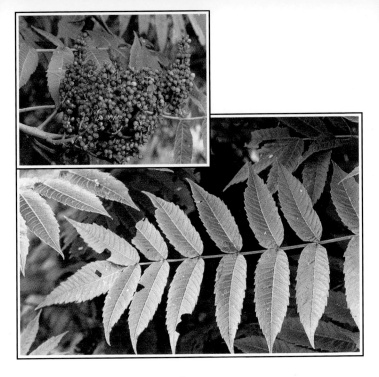

# Smooth Sumac
*Rhus glabra*

**Also Called:** Scarlet Sumac, Shoemake

**Description:** Sumac is a shrub that can grow as tall as 15 feet.

*Leaves:* Leaves grow from 1 to 3 feet long and are composed of 10 to 30 leaflets. Growing opposite each other along a smooth stem, these leaflets are 2 to 4 inches long, 141 slender and pointed, with toothed edges.

*Flowers:* Greenish-yellow flowers bloom in clusters at the ends of branches and produce clusters of small, round, bright red berries. These berries are covered with a very fine hair.

**Where:** Smooth Sumac grows in old fields, thickets, power line right of ways, pastures, and along the roadsides over much of the United States. It ranges from Arizona and Colorado, eastward to Maine and south to Florida.

**What:** Harvest leaves, root bark, and tree bark.

**When:** Sumac leaves are harvested during the growing season from May to June or July, while they are green in color.

Root and tree bark are harvested in the spring and fall. Bark is most easily harvested in the spring when the sap is rising. Never girdle the branches, but strip bark from one side only.

Care needs to be taken around power line right of ways where herbicides may have been sprayed. Do not harvest any plants from an area that has been sprayed. These plants will contain harmful residues.

| **How:** | See Page 11-12 for general guidelines on cleaning, drying, and preparing leaves and bark for market. |
| | Dry the leaves out of the sun. Leaves should remain green when they dry. |
| | Be sure to keep root bark and tree bark separate. The root bark stops at the top of the soil. Above that point is tree bark. |
| **Uses:** | Sumac leaves are used to treat asthma and other respiratory ailments. Fruits are used as a gargle for sore throats and sores in the mouth, and as a tea for fevers. |

## Notes

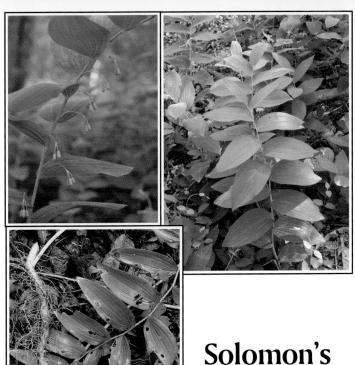

# Solomon's Seal

*Polygonatum biflorum*

**Also Called:** Seal Root, Dropberry

**Description:** This perennial plant grows from 1 to 3 feet in height. The stem often curves like a bow as it grows, with the tips of the stems arching up and then over toward the earth.

*Leaves:* Leaves are large, often up to 4 inches in length, and grow alternately along the stem. The leaves hang down from the stem, hiding the flowers, which hang in pairs from the crook of the leaves.

*Flowers:* The flowers are greenish-white, bell-shaped, and hang along the stem, underneath the leaves. (Note: You can tell the difference between Solomon's Seal and False Solomon's Seal by where the flowers and berries grow. The flowers and berries of False Solomon's Seal are found at the end of the stem, while those of Solomon's Seal grow along the under side of the stem.)

*Fruit:* Flowers are followed by green berries that ripen to a blue-black color.

*Roots:* The root is yellowish-white when dug and bears scars along the top where old stems once grew. The roots are long with many hair rootlets on the under side.

**Where:** Solomon's Seal grows in moist, rich, shady woods and is often found growing with Bloodroot and Mayapple. It ranges from Connecticut south to Florida, west to Texas and Wisconsin.

**What:** Harvest the roots.

**When:** The roots of Solomon's Seal are harvested in the fall after the seed has set. Roots are long, so be sure to dig carefully to get the entire root. Leave at least 25% of the patch to regenerate for future harvests.

**How:** See Pages 10-11 for general guidelines on cleaning, drying, and preparing roots for market.

Rinsing Solomon's Seal roots in running water is a good way to loosen dirt that clings to the root hairs. Rinse thoroughly until water runs clear. Solomon's Seal roots dry very slowly, so slicing this root lengthwise will help speed the drying process.

**Uses:** Used externally to treat cuts, bruises, sores, poison ivy, and other skin rashes. Has also been used traditionally for arthritis, rheumatism, indigestion, and respiratory problems.

## Notes

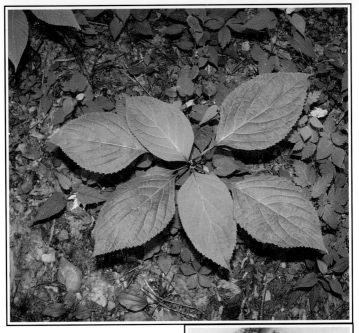

# Stone Root
*Collinsonia Canadensis*

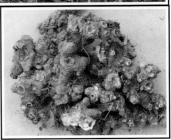

**Also Called:** Knob Root, Horse Balm, Richweed, Ox-Balm, Citronella Horse Balm

**Description:** Stone Root is another aromatic member of the mint family. Both the leaves and flowers have a tangy 149

lemon or citronella-like scent. Stone Root grows up to 4 feet tall on stout, square, branched stems.

*Leaves:* Leaves are opposite and grow from 3 to 8 inches long. They vary from oval to oblong and may occasionally be heart-shaped at the base. Leaves at the base of the plant have slender stems and are larger than the upper, almost stemless leaves.

*Flowers:* Stone Root blooms mid to late summer. Its pale yellow funnel-shaped flowers split at the end into an upper and lower lip, the lower one being larger than the upper and fringed. Long stamens reach well past the edges of the lips.

*Roots:* Stone Root lives up to its name. Fresh or dry, these roots are incredibly hard. They grow horizontally and are thick and woody. The upper surface is knotty with scars from previous stems.

**Where:** Stone Root grows in rich woods and moist, shady ravines. It ranges from Canada to Wisconsin south to Florida to Kansas and Missouri.

**What:** Harvest the roots. **Stone Root is considered an endangered species in**

**the state of Wisconsin.** It is protected by federal and state governments elsewhere. Ask your State Plant Board, State Agriculture Department, or county agriculture agent for their guidelines and laws.

**When:** Harvest roots in the fall when plant growth has stopped and the seeds have matured.

**How:** See Page 10-11 for general guidelines on cleaning, drying, and preparing roots for market.

Stone Root can be cut or sliced to speed drying time. Dry the roots in a well ventilated area and keep the air moving around the roots.

**Cultivation:** Because wild Stone Root is a protected or endangered plant in some states, one would be wise to consider cultivating it. Under the right conditions, Stone Root is not difficult to grow and is sometimes even grown as an ornamental plant. Growing conditions should duplicate those of the plants natural habitat – moist acidic soil and dappled shade being essential to success. Seeds can be sown outdoors in late fall or early spring. Germination takes 8 to 10 weeks. Seedlings can be transplanted when they're large enough to handle. Roots should not be harvested until the third year or later.

**Uses:** Traditionally Stone Root has been used in bladder and kidney ailments as well as for heart disease, hemorrhoids, and varicose veins. It also functions as a diuretic.

## Notes

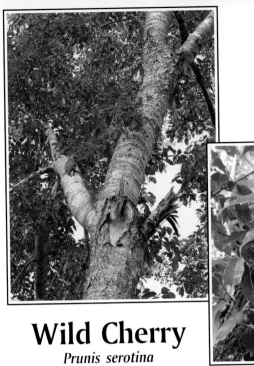

# Wild Cherry
*Prunis serotina*

**Also Called:** Black Cherry, Mountain Black Cherry, Rum or Whiskey Cherry

**Description:** When growing in optimal conditions, Wild Cherry is a tall stately tree with a straight trunk that can reach to 100 feet in height. The trunk is clear of branches for up to 30 feet and can grow to a diameter of 4 to 5 feet. Under less than optimal conditions, Wild Cherry is medium-height and poorly formed.

*Leaves:* Oval to oblong lance-shaped, thick leaves are 2 to 5 inches long and 1 to 1½ inches wide. They are alternate and finely serrated on the edges. Leaves are smooth on both sides, dark shiny green above and pale green below.

*Flowers:* In the spring, before the leaves have fully formed, long drooping clusters of white flowers bloom. The clusters measure 4 to 6 inches, and the flowers are 5-petaled.

*Fruit:* The flowers are followed by clusters of pea-sized cherries that ripen in the early fall. They are reddish black and have a purple juicy pulp which is bitter sweet in taste. The cherries are food for song birds, who distribute the seed far and wide.

*Bark:* Wild Cherry bark is rough and black on older trees and smooth and flecked with narrow horizontal bands of small pores called *lenticels* on young trees. Bark on branches is smooth, turning from pale green or bronze to a bright red or dark brown as they age.

**Where:** Wild Cherry grows in a wide range of habitats from dry woods, wastelands, and pastures to roadsides, fence rows, and creek bottoms. It grows best in deep rich soil with adequate moisture. It ranges throughout the eastern states from Maine to Minnesota, and south to eastern Texas and central Florida.

**What:**
Both "thick" and "thin" bark. Thick cherry bark is the bark taken from the trunk or older branches of the mature part of the tree. It is generally ¼ to ½ inch thick. Thin cherry bark is taken from new growth and the younger limbs of the tree. This bark is generally only an eighth of an inch think.

**When:**
Bark is best harvested in early spring, before the sap rises.

**How:**
See Page 10 for general guidelines for harvesting barks, and Page 12 for drying and preparing for market.

Take bark from only one side of the branches or the trunk. Never girdle the trunk or the branches as this will kill the tree.

**Uses:**
Wild Cherry bark has a long history of use for respiratory problems and is the source for the well-known Wild Cherry cough syrup. Used to treat coughs, colds, fevers, sore throats, bronchitis, and pneumonia, Wild Cherry has a soothing and sedative

effect on the nervous system.
The cherries are a rich source
of vitamin C.

## <u>Notes</u>

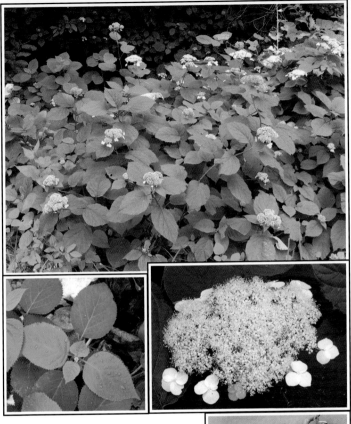

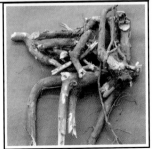

# Wild Hydrangea

*Hydrangea arborescens*

**Also Called:** Smooth Hydrangea, Seven Barks

**Description:** Hydrangea is a perennial shrub that is formed by numerous unbranched vigorous canes. The canes have a rough bark that peels off in several thin layers, each of a different color, giving it the common name Seven Barks. Hydrangea grows 5 to 6 feet or more in height and has a spread of 3 to 5 feet.

*Leaves:* Leaves are oval or sometimes heart-shaped. They are broad, opposite, and sharply toothed. The upper surface is a smooth, dull, dark green and the lower slightly paler and sometimes hairy.

*Flowers:* Showy flat-topped clusters of small flowers bloom from late spring continuing into early summer. Flowers turn from green to white and then to brown and continue on the plant throughout the summer. Larger papery-white sterile flowers are often present along the edge of the cluster. Sometimes Hydrangea will bloom a second time in the early fall.

*Roots:* Roots vary in length and are roughly branched. They are white and smooth and covered with a thin pale yellow or light brown bark that easily peels away. When fresh the roots are juicy and can be easily cut. When dry they become very tough and hard. The root itself is tasteless, but the root bark has a sweet somewhat pungent taste.

**Where:** Wild Hydrangea grows in rich woods, on rocky slopes, and on stream banks. It ranges from New York to Missouri and Oklahoma, south to Northern Florida, Georgia, Mississippi, Arkansas, and Louisiana.

**What:** Harvest the roots.

**When:** Roots are harvested in the fall, after the plant has gone to seed.

**How:** See Pages 10-11 for general guidelines on cleaning, drying, and preparing roots for market.

Because Hydrangea root becomes very tough when dried, it is best to cut the root in short pieces while it is freshly dug and still pliable.

**Uses:** Traditionally used to treat bladder and kidney problems including kidney stones. Also used as a diuretic.

## Notes

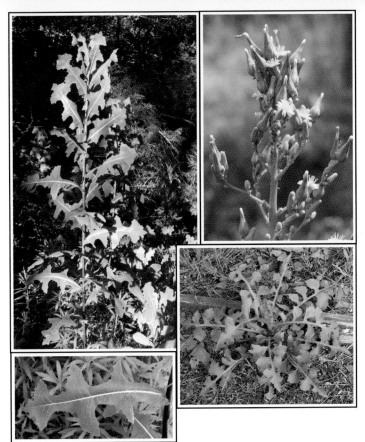

# Wild Lettuce
*Lactuca canadensis*

**Also Called:** Tall Lettuce, Horseweed, Canada Lettuce, Wild Opium

**Description:** Wild Lettuce is a tall annual or biennial plant. Usually the plant is over 30 inches tall and can grow to

10 feet or better. The stem is erect, smooth, green or reddish in color with a whitish film and produces a white milky juice when crushed.

*Leaves:* Leaves are long and vary from lance-shaped to deeply lobed similar to dandelion leaves. They are medium green in color, flimsy in texture, and have no stalk.

*Flowers:* Small yellow flowers bloom in clusters on loosely branched stalks. The flowers resemble very small dandelion flowers and bloom from early summer through early fall.

**Where:** Wild Lettuce grows in clearings, fields, fencerows, and thickets throughout the United States. It thrives in low damp places.

**What:** Harvest entire above-ground part of this plant.

**When:** Harvest Wild Lettuce in the summer or early fall when the plant is in bloom.

**How:** See pages 11-12 for general guidelines on cleaning, drying, and preparing herbs for market.

It is best to collect and dry wild lettuce during periods of dry weather.

Shredding or cutting the stems and leaves will speed drying time.

**Uses:** Traditionally Wild Lettuce has been used as a mild sedative and nerve tonic to calm restlessness and anxiety and to induce sleep. The milky juice from the stems has been used for skin irritations including poison ivy rash and warts. Because the milky juice from the plant becomes firm and brown when exposed to the air and resembles opium in look and smell, Wild Lettuce has gained an undeserved reputation as an opium substitute.

When young and tender, Wild Lettuce leaves are an excellent addition to salads and can also be cooked as a potherb. The leaves are rich in vitamins and iron.

### Notes

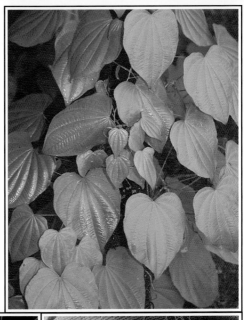

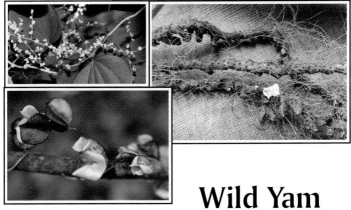

# Wild Yam
*Dioscorea villosa*

**Also Called:** Colic Root, Rheumatism Root, China Root, Devil's Bones

**Description:** Wild Yam is a perennial vine that grows from 5 to 15 feet, twining over bushes, trees, and fences. The stem is slender, smooth, rarely branches, and generally twines in a counterclockwise direction.

*Leaves:* Wild Yam leaves rise on long slender stems. Leaf placement on the stem varies. At the base leaves may be found in whorls of 3 to 8. Leaves in the middle portion of the stem are nearly opposite, while upper leaves are alternate. The leaves are heart-shaped with 7 to 11 very distinct veins running from the stem end to the tip of the leaf. The underside is downy and grayish in color.

*Flowers:* Small greenish-yellow flowers bloom in drooping loose clusters from mid-spring to early summer.

*Fruit:* The fruit is an oval 3-celled, 3-winged yellowish-green pod. When it ripens in the fall, the pod turns brown and opens along the winged angles, dispersing the seeds. The dried pods remain on the stem throughout much of the winter and are easily used for plant identification.

*Roots:* Wild Yam roots grow horizontally beneath the surface of the soil. They are knobby and have numerous tangled feeders. Dried Wild Yam is notoriously tough, impossible to cut, and difficult to grind.

**Where:** Wild Yam grows in moist, wet thickets, roadsides, swamps, and hardwood forests. It is found in eastern North America and ranges from southern Canada and New England west to Wisconsin and south from Texas to Tennessee. It is more commonly found in the south.

**What:** Harvest the roots.

**When:** Roots are harvested in the fall, after the seeds have set.

**How:** See Pages 10-11 for general guidelines on cleaning, drying, and preparing roots for market.

Wild Yam roots do not grow deep, but run horizontally under the ground, sometimes to a length of 2 feet or more. Care should be taken to disentangle other roots and debris from the numerous feeder roots.

**Uses:** Traditionally used for colic, indigestion, liver problems, and asthma.

Many people mistakenly believe

that Wild Yam contains progesterone, a hormone used to treat menopausal discomforts. Wild Yam contains diosgenin, a saponin that is used in chemically creating synthetic progesterone and steroids used to treat asthma, arthritis, and eczema.

Other synthetic products produced from Wild Yam include human sex hormones (birth control pills) and drugs to treat menopause, PMS, and impotency.

## Notes

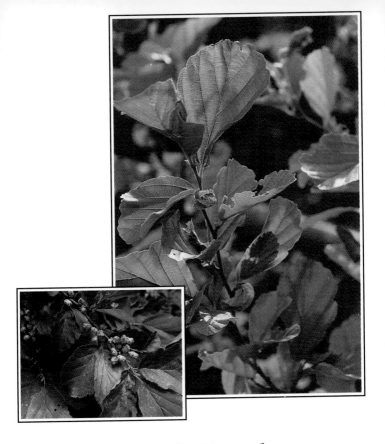

# Witch Hazel
### *Hamamelis virginiana*

**Also Called:** Snapping Hazel, Long Boughs, Spotted Alder, Tobacco Wood, Winterbloom

**Description:** Witch Hazel is a small tree growing from 5 to 15 feet in height. The trunk is often crooked or 169

twisted, and its branches forked and smooth. Witch Hazel bark is a brownish grey in color.

*Leaves:* Witch Hazel leaves are round to oval in shape and are thick and wavy. Their edges are toothed.

*Flowers:* Unlike most plants, Witch Hazel flowers in the fall, after its leaves are gone. From September to November its pale yellow flowers blossom along the branches. The flower has very thin, threadlike petals that twist and curl around themselves as they grow.

*Fruit:* The fruit stays on the tree through the winter and matures into seed pods the following summer. When the seed pods burst, the seeds are thrown out, sometimes flying many feet away from the tree.

**Where:** Witch Hazel grows in light woods that range from moist to dry, usually on the borders of forests and on rocky stream banks. It ranges over most of the eastern United States.

**What:** Harvest the leaves and bark.

**When:** The leaves are harvested in the summer and fall, the bark in the spring and fall. The leaves grow on a short stalk and can be harvested without damaging the branches of the tree. The bark is most easily harvested in the spring when the sap is rising. When harvesting tree bark, take it from the branches of the tree, and from only one side of each branch you harvest.

**How:**      See Page 11-12 for general guidelines on cleaning, drying, and preparing leaves and bark for market.

**Uses:**      Soothing to cuts, bruises, sprains, insect bites, burns, and sunburns. Witch Hazel has also been used to control internal and external bleeding, and to treat aching joints and sore muscles.

## Notes

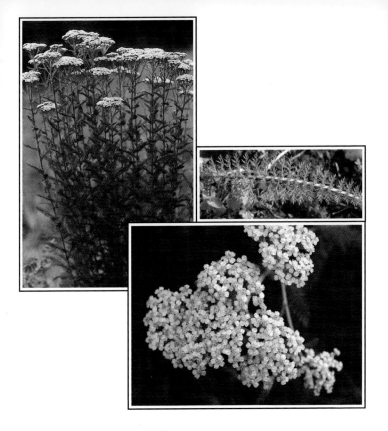

# Yarrow
*Achillea millefolium*

**Also Called:** Milfoil, Thousand Leaf, Soldier's Woundwort, Carpenter's Weed

**Description:** Yarrow is a perennial, upright plant that grows from 1 to 3 feet in height with feathery, fern-like leaves and a flat-topped flower head.

*Leaves:* Yarrow leaves are dark green and grow 3 to 4 inches long and an inch or so across. They are shaped like a feather, and each segment of the leaf is also shaped like a feather. They grow alternately along the stem.

*Flowers:* Individual flowers are small but they gather together in showy flat-topped clusters. They are a dull white or occasionally pink. Each flower has 5 petals that are wider than they are long and are toothed at the end. Yarrow flowers from late spring to early fall.

**Where:** Yarrow is a common wayside herb that grows throughout most of North America. It can be found along road-sides, in fields, and waste places.

**What:** Harvest the entire above-ground part of the plant including stem, leaves, and flower.

**When:** Harvest when the plant is in bloom.

**How:** See Pages 11-12 for general guidelines on cleaning, drying, and preparing herbs for market. It is best to cut the plant off above the ground, leaving the root system intact. Be sure to remove any excess debris that may become entangled in the leaves and flower clusters. It is wise to leave at least 25%

of any patch unharvested.

**Cultivation:** Yarrow can be grown easily from seed, or you can propagate by root division in the early spring or fall. Yarrow does best in full sun and is not picky about soil, as long as it's well drained. Once planted, Yarrow will spread, so take care in choosing where you plant this herb.

**Uses:** Over the centuries Yarrow has been used for just about every ailment known to man. Most notably it has been used for treating wounds. Yarrow contains alkaloids that help blood to clot. Yarrow has also been a popular remedy for colds and flu as it promotes sweating, functions as an expectorant, and reduces pain. It is effective in alleviating gastric inflammation and other digestive disorders including food poisoning, vomiting, and dry heaves.

## Notes

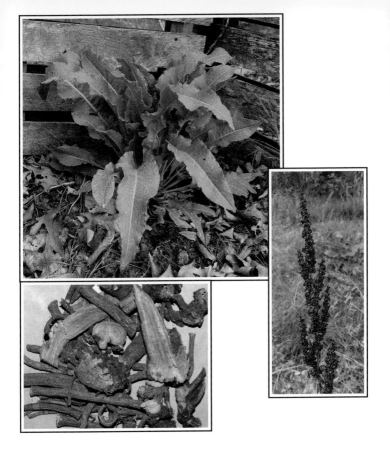

# Yellow or Curly Dock
### *Rumex crispus*

**Also Called:** Narrow Dock, Sour Dock, Common Dock, Garden Patience

**Description:** Yellow Dock is a perennial plant growing 2 to 5 feet in height with narrow lance-shaped leaves and erect flowering stalks.

*Leaves:* Leaves are lance-shaped, narrow, and grow 6 to 12 inches long. They are wavy or curly on the edges, giving rise to the name Curly Dock.

*Flowers:* Flowers appear in mid-summer in long dense clusters along the stem. They are yellow to green early, turning rose and red or red brown in the fall. Brown seed heads remain on the plant into the winter.

*Roots:* Yellow Dock roots are large, spindle shaped, and fleshy. They can grow 2 to 3 inches thick at the top and 8 to 12 inches long with few or no rootlets. The root bark is thick and dark brown in color and the inside is a rich yellow.

**Where:** Yellow Dock is found throughout the United States along roadsides, in grassy places, cultivated fields, waste ground, and disturbed sites.

**What:** Harvest the root.

**When:** Roots are harvested in the late summer or early fall after the flowering tops have turned brown.

Many consider Yellow Dock a noxious weed and would welcome its removal from their property.

**How:**     See Pages 10-11 for general guidelines on cleaning, drying, and preparing roots for market

Roots are exceedingly difficult to pull up and must be dug from the ground. After washing, Yellow Dock roots can be dried whole or split lengthwise in half or quarters. Be sure roots are thoroughly dry before storing in paper or burlap bags.

**Cultivation:**     Although many would resist the idea of cultivating a plant considered an invasive weed, Yellow Dock is easy to grow from seed and requires little care. It prefers a sunny well drained location. To prevent its tendency to aggressively spread, harvest the roots every fall. The seed heads are also used by crafters who make wreaths and dried arrangements.

**Uses:**     Traditionally used as a blood cleanser and purifier. Yellow Dock is well known for its ability to increase the amount of iron available to the blood system, to cleanse the lymph system, and to aid in chronic skin diseases.

Caution is advised as large doses can cause gastric upset, diarrhea, or nausea.

The leaves of Yellow Dock have long been gathered as a spring green or potherb. The young greens are a rich source of vitamins A and C. They are best gathered throughout the winter and in the very early spring with the nights are still cold and the days cool.

## Notes